Facilitated Stretching

THIRD EDITION

Robert E. McAtee | Jeff Charland

Human Kinetics

Library of Congress Cataloging-in-Publication Data

McAtee, Robert E., 1948-
  Facilitated stretching / Robert E. McAtee. -- 3rd ed.
    p. cm.
  Includes bibliographical references and index.
  ISBN-13: 978-0-7360-6248-0 (soft cover)
  ISBN-10: 0-7360-6248-3 (soft cover)
  1. Stretching exercises--Popular works.   2. Athletes.   3. Physical therapy--Popular
works.   I. Title.
    RA781.63.M33 2007
    613.7'1--dc22
                                          2006037979

ISBN-10: 0-7360-6248-3
ISBN-13: 978-0-7360-6248-0

Art on page 4 adapted from J.H. Wilmore and D.L. Costill, 2004, *Physiology of Sport and Exercise, Third Edition* (Champaign, IL: Human Kinetics). Art on pages 20, 21, 38, 48, 51, 54, 58, 61, 68, 72, 82, 83, 90, 95, 97, 110, 111, 119, and 120 adapted from R.S. Behnke, *Kinetic Anatomy, Second Edition* (Champaign, IL: Human Kinetics) from pages 178, 216, and 13; 178; 180; 202; 183; 198; 178; 202; 216; 216 and 217; 51 and 50; 47; 13 and 47; 81 and 84; 81 and 84; 132 and 129; 130; 135; 135 and 132; respectively.

Acquisitions Editor: Loarn D. Robertson, PhD; **Reviewer:** Keith Eric Grant; **Developmental Editor:** Maggie Schwarzentraub; **Assistant Editor:** Maureen Eckstein; **Copyeditor:** Joyce Sexton; **Proofreader:** Pam Johnson; **Indexer:** Betty Frizzéll; **Permission Manager:** Carly Breeding; **Graphic Designer:** Bob Reuther; **Graphic Artist:** Yvonne Griffith; **Cover Designer:** Keith Blomberg; **Photographer (cover and interior):** Joe Jovanovich; **Art Manager:** Kelly Hendren; **Illustrators:** Jason M. McAlexander, MFA, and Mic Greenberg (figure 1.1 only); **Printer:** United Graphics Inc.

Printed in the United States of America   10 9 8 7 6 5 4 3

Human Kinetics
Web site: www.HumanKinetics.com

United States: Human Kinetics
P.O. Box 5076
Champaign, IL 61825-5076
800-747-4457
e-mail: humank@hkusa.com

Canada: Human Kinetics
475 Devonshire Road, Unit 100
Windsor, ON N8Y 2L5
800-465-7301 (in Canada only)
e-mail: info@hkcanada.com

Europe: Human Kinetics
107 Bradford Road
Stanningley
Leeds LS28 6AT, United Kingdom
+44 (0)113 255 5665
e-mail: hk@hkeurope.com

Australia: Human Kinetics
57A Price Avenue
Lower Mitcham, South Australia 5062
08 8372 0999
e-mail: info@hkaustralia.com

New Zealand: Human Kinetics
Division of Sports Distributors NZ Ltd.
P.O. Box 300 226 Albany
North Shore City, Auckland
0064 9 448 1207
e-mail: info@humankinetics.co.nz

To my wife, Treeanna MacHardy, whose love and support have been instrumental from the beginning.

CONTENTS

PREFACE

Welcome to the third edition of *Facilitated Stretching*. Like its predecessors, this book has been shaped by thousands of readers and seminar participants who have made suggestions, submitted stretches, or asked tough questions that made us go find answers.

Facilitated stretching is an easy way to maintain or improve flexibility and coordination. If you're a sport therapist, athletic trainer, sport physician, coach, or competitive athlete, you'll find valuable information here for optimizing performance. Whether you're an accomplished athlete or are just beginning a fitness program, you'll find that these techniques will help you gain increased flexibility and coordination, which can help prevent injuries and improve your enjoyment of your chosen activities.

In this third edition, you'll find over 80 stretches, including 13 new or modified partner-assisted stretches and 19 new or modified self-stretches. You'll also notice a brand-new feature: Descriptions of strengthening exercises for use with the spiral patterns of PNF (proprioceptive neuromuscular facilitation). You'll find a total of 16 tables, 35 line drawings, and 350 photographs illustrating these stretches and strengthening exercises, which are based on our experience teaching this technique to thousands of people over the last 15 years. We've incorporated your feedback to make this method easier to understand and more effective. To this end, we've reorganized the book to make it easier to use. Like its predecessor, this edition also emphasizes your independence by teaching you to do these exercises on your own.

The book is organized into three parts, with each part containing three chapters.

In part I, chapter 1, we discuss general guidelines for any type of stretching, including the importance of using good biomechanics. Then, in chapter 2, we provide a detailed description of facilitated stretching. In chapter 3, we take a close look at the spiral–diagonal patterns of PNF and how we use them in facilitated stretching to improve flexibility and the interaction of synergistic groups of muscles. New in this edition are examples in this chapter of strength training work using the spiral patterns, incorporating stability balls and elastic bands.

In part II, we show you, step by step, how to stretch the major muscles, both singly and in groups. Chapter 4 covers the hips and legs; chapter 5 is devoted to the shoulders and arms; and chapter 6 details stretches for the neck and torso.

In part III, we offer what we consider to be more advanced work. In chapter 7, we expand on the topic of combining stretching and soft tissue work. This chapter now includes a broader discussion of conditions that respond to a blend of manual therapy techniques and facilitated stretching, including work on the hamstrings, hip abductors, piriformis, rotator cuff, scalenes, and serratus anterior.

Because of numerous requests from readers and seminar participants, in chapter 8 we added stretching routines for a variety of activities, including running, throwing and racket sports, cycling, golf, swimming, everyday stretches, and "rusty hinges" routines.

In chapter 9, we categorize some common soft tissue problems associated with popular athletic activities and suggest some appropriate stretching and strengthening exercises to improve your "game." We provide general guidelines and a home treatment program you can use to care for some minor problems or even prevent them from occurring. If you've suffered from nagging "aches and pains" with certain activities, these exercises may be beneficial for you.

As an added bonus and valuable learning tool, we include with the book, on the inside back cover, a 90-minute DVD that clearly demonstrates selected stretches and strengthening exercises. The DVD allows us to give you more detail than the book alone can. Stretches and exercises illustrated on the DVD are identified by the icon shown at the left. You'll find a complete list of the DVD stretces and exercises on page 184.

A second bonus feature, for teachers who adopt the book as a classroom text, is free access to an online test package. The package includes test questions in several formats (multiple choice, true or false, fill in the blank). Instructors can create print versions of their own tests by selecting from the question pool; create, store, and retrieve their own questions; select their own test forms and save them for later editing or printing; or export the tests into a word processing program.

We remind you that before starting any exercise or fitness program, prudent readers will consult with their physicians. We've taken care to ensure that the information given in this text is accurate; but medical knowledge is constantly changing, and as new information becomes available, changes in treatment, equipment, and procedures become necessary.

We hope the collective knowledge we have distilled into these pages will be a valuable addition to your active lifestyle.

ACKNOWLEDGMENTS

No book can be written and produced without the help of many people.

First of all, I want to thank Dave Charland. After his brother Jeff's untimely death, Dave graciously agreed to co-author Chapter 9, our new material on routines for dealing with soft-tissue injuries. Without his enthusiastic participation, this information would never have made it into the book.

Dave Morgan of the United Kingdom, a careful reader indeed, noticed two errors in the second edition, now corrected, in the muscle table describing the rhomboids.

Greg Gebben, understanding the importance of music in feeding the creative process, gifted me with a 5-CD set of "Music for the Mozart Effect," with music to enhance creativity, focus, strength, relaxation, and healing. I needed all 5 discs throughout the production of this book!

On a similar note, I had the opportunity to spend a week in Hawaii, where I was able to devote eight hours a day to writing. I spent the bulk of those hours listening to traditional Hawaiian music on the radio. After I got home and continued to write, I could recreate the musical ambience of that week (even deep in the Colorado winter) with the help of www.hawaiianrainbow.com, which streams Hawaiian music 24 hours a day, seven days a week.

Thanks to Leon Chaitow, Roger Enoka, and Gordon Chalmers for their assistance in understanding and incorporating information on the role of reflexes in stretching. Of course, any errors in the manuscript are mine alone.

Thanks to Loarn Robertson, PhD, acquisitions editor at Human Kinetics. He guided me through the early stages of the manuscript, helping to shape and focus it.

I thoroughly enjoyed working with Maggie Schwarzentraub, developmental editor, ably assisted by Maureen Eckstein. Their organizational skills and creativity have made this the best editing experience of my writing career. They took into account my teaching and travel schedule in setting manuscript deadlines, scheduling the photo and video shoots, and handling the myriad details that went into the production of this book.

Joe Jovanovich made shooting 1,000 photos in two days seem easy, and Doug Fink and his crew maintained a relaxed and easy atmosphere during our video shoot.

Many thanks to our models—Rebekah Hopkins, Abraham Jones, and Kia Locksley. They worked long hours and managed to stay upbeat and positive, and they were always willing to take "just one more shot."

I'd also like to thank the rest of the Human Kinetics family who have a hand in the development, production, and marketing of the book.

Bob McAtee

In memory of Jeff Charland, my brother and mentor. I had the great fortune of working with Jeff for 17 years in the field, as a physical therapy assistant, athletic trainer, and, more recently, as a physical therapist. Thank you, brother, for all the opportunities and achievements you have shared with me; you are a big part of who I am. Thanks to Bob McAtee and Human Kinetics for allowing me to carry on the Charland participation in this book.

David Charland

PART I

The Prerequisites

In this part, we discuss some general guidelines for any kind of stretching (chapter 1), then provide a detailed description of facilitated stretching (chapter 2). In chapter 3, we take a close look at the spiral–diagonal patterns of proprioceptive neuromuscular facilitation (PNF) and explain how they are used in facilitated stretching to improve the interaction of synergistic groups of muscles. This includes using the patterns for strengthening exercises as well as for stretching.

Understanding the Basics of Stretching

In this chapter we'll look at some of the principles of stretching, including the types of muscle contractions, stretch reflexes, and some of the different techniques of stretching. Chapter 2 presents a more complete discussion of facilitated stretching.

Types of Muscle Contractions

Two types of muscle contractions, isotonic and isometric, are of special interest to us in our discussion of stretching.

An isotonic contraction is a voluntary muscle contraction that causes movement. There are two types of isotonic contractions: concentric contraction, in which the muscle shortens as it works, and eccentric contraction, in which the muscle resists while being lengthened by an outside force. For example, a concentric isotonic contraction of the biceps brachii muscle happens when you bend your elbow, as in doing an arm curl with dumbbells (figure 1.1, p. 4). You perform an eccentric contraction of the biceps as you lower the dumbbells. In this case, the outside force being resisted is a combination of gravity and the weight of the dumbbells. An eccentric contraction is also called negative work.

An isometric contraction is a voluntary contraction in which no movement occurs. When you hold a dumbbell in midcurl, you're doing an isometric contraction.

Reflexes Relevant to Stretching

According to most anatomy and physiology textbooks, a reflex is an automatic, involuntary response to a stimulus. In the last few years, the scientific and research communities have reached a broad consensus that reflexes are much more complex, and not as automatic as previously believed. In many cases, the effect of a reflex is task dependent (Hultborn, 2001). This new knowledge of reflexes has a significant effect on our explanations of why various forms of stretching work, including facilitated stretching. We discuss this more in each section below.

Myotatic Stretch Reflex

In general, the myotatic stretch reflex prevents a muscle from stretching too far too fast, which helps protect the joint from injury. This reflex is what you see when a physician tests your reflexes. She strikes your biceps tendon with a small rubber hammer, and your arm automatically bends at the elbow. Proprioceptors in the biceps, called "muscle spindles," monitor the length and tension of the muscle. When the muscle

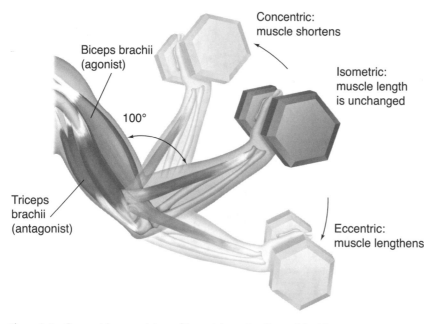

Concentric:
muscle shortens

Isometric:
muscle length
is unchanged

Biceps brachii
(agonist)

100°

Triceps
brachii
(antagonist)

Eccentric:
muscle lengthens

Figure 1.1 Concentric, eccentric, and isometric contractions of the biceps.

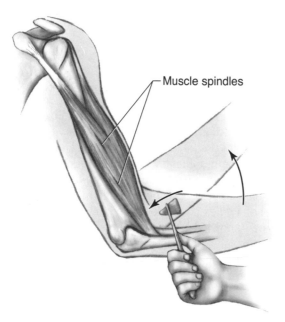

Muscle spindles

Figure 1.2 A representation of the muscle spindles, which mediate the myotatic stretch eflex.

lengthens too quickly, as happens when the reflex hammer strikes the tendon, the muscle spindles are stimulated and reflexively cause the muscle to contract, which causes the arm to bend. This reflexive contraction, the stretch reflex, prevents overstretching of the elbow joint and the biceps (figure 1.2).

The stretch reflex may be strong, weak, or absent, depending on the situation. Whether the reflex is initiated depends on a number of conditions, including the speed and distance the muscle is stretched, whether the stretch is occurring because the opposing muscle is contracting, or if the opposing muscle is inactive, as in the hammer reflex example given previously.

Inverse Stretch Reflex

As described in most textbooks, the inverse stretch reflex (also called autogenic inhibition) is mediated by stretch receptors called Golgi tendon organs (GTOs), which are located in the musculotendinous junction and the tendon. Traditional PNF theory includes discussion of the inverse stretch reflex and its supposed effects following an isometric contraction. The common belief has been that GTOs monitor the load on the tendon. If the load becomes too great, the GTOs are stimulated. In turn, they were thought to cause the muscle to relax through neurological inhibition.

It seems clear now that while the GTOs do monitor muscle tension, they do not mediate the inverse stretch reflex, if such a reflex even exists. Scientists are still trying to understand the GTOs and believe that their effect is task-dependent, and may inhibit or excite the muscle in which they're located, as well as affecting neighboring muscles. As we said earlier, reflexes are much more complex than previously explained.

Reciprocal Innervation

Sir Charles Sherrington's research in the early to mid-1900s helped develop a model for how the neuromuscular system operates (Sherrington 1947). The textbook explanation of his law of reciprocal innervation (also called reciprocal inhibition) has described a reflex loop mediated by the muscle spindles. When a muscle contracts, reciprocal inhibition was thought to inhibit the opposing muscle. This inhibition would allow movement to occur around a joint. For instance, when the quadriceps muscle contracts, the hamstrings would be reciprocally inhibited, thereby allowing the knee to straighten. If this reflex loop is not functioning well, the muscles could be fighting each other, and the movement might become difficult or be compromised (figure 1.3).

Although reciprocal inhibition can be seen under experimental conditions, in real life it is much more complex. It is more likely to occur when necessary, as

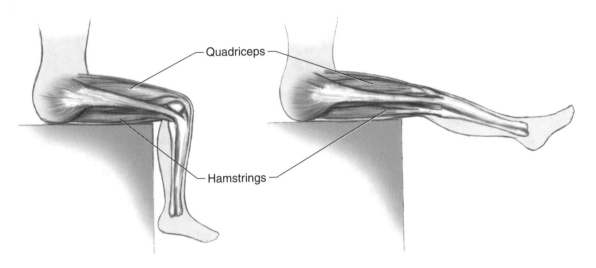

Figure 1.3 **Reciprocal inhibition. When the quadriceps contract, the hamstrings may be inhibited, allowing the knee to straighten easily.**

during joint movement, and not occur when undesirable, as in joint stabilization, when we need to have opposing muscles cocontracting. Reflexes are now seen as task-dependent, not as automatic, involuntary reactions that always occur the same way.

Types of Stretching

Stretching can be broadly categorized as passive, active, or assisted. Some of these categories can be further subdivided, based on their movement characteristics, into ballistic, dynamic, and static. Many styles of stretching are used today, some of which are variations developed for specific sports or activities.

Passive Stretching

Passive stretching is done to the stretcher by a partner; it can be ballistic or static. In a passive stretch, the stretcher relaxes and the partner moves the limb being stretched to gain new range of motion (ROM) (figure 1.4).

Passive stretching is often used to increase flexibility at the extremes of ROM, as in gymnastics, where maximum flexibility is crucial for performance. It may also be used when active movement causes pain.

Done carelessly or with poor form, passive stretching can cause muscle injury because the partner assisting the stretching cannot feel the sensations of the stretcher and may overstretch the

muscle. Passive stretching requires proper training and good communication between the stretcher and the partner.

Active and Active-Assisted Stretching

Active stretching means that the stretcher is doing the work instead of having a partner do it. Active forms of stretching are generally considered safer than passive stretching because the chance of overstretching and causing injury are greatly reduced when the stretcher controls the force and duration of the stretch.

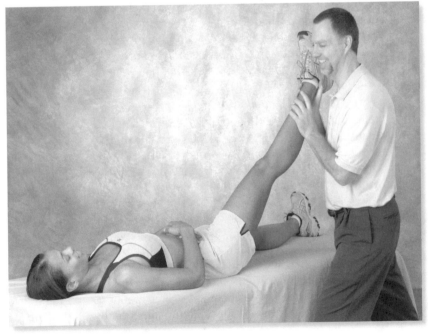

Figure 1.4 **Passive stretching is done to the stretcher by a partner.**

Active-assisted stretching combines active movement by the stretcher with help from a partner, either to add passive stretch or to provide resistance to motion, thus blending active and passive stretching types. Facilitated stretching falls into this category, as do a number of other techniques, such as those described next.

MUSCLE ENERGY TECHNIQUE

Another form of active-assisted stretching is "muscle energy technique" (MET), a technique that developed in osteopathy about the same time that proprioceptive neuromuscular facilitation (PNF) was evolving in physical therapy. According to Chaitow (2001, p.1), MET "targets the soft tissues primarily, although it also makes a major contribution towards joint mobilisation. . . ." Like PNF techniques, MET uses an isometric contraction of the target muscle before the stretch. Muscle energy technique, however, uses only minimal force during the isometric phase. The stretch is most often done passively. Because MET developed in osteopathic medicine, its primary goal is joint mobilization, which is not a goal of PNF techniques.

Some variations or refinements of MET include the following:

■ *The Lewit technique (PIR)*—Dr. Karel Lewit, a Czech neurologist, refers to his method as PIR, or "postisometric relaxation," referring to the decreased resistance of a muscle to stretch following its isometric contraction (Lewit, 1999). PIR was thought to be a form of autogenic inhibition, mediated by the GTOs, but that premise has been abandoned for the same reasons we outlined above. Lewit's technique focuses on relaxing hypertonic muscles to reduce pain; and any increase in ROM occurs because more slack has been achieved in the tissue, not because of stretching.

■ *Reciprocal inhibition stretching (RI)*—Reciprocal inhibition refers to a neurological reflex that may cause one muscle to relax when its opposing muscle contracts. RI stretching is used to stretch a target muscle by first contracting the opposing muscle. This contraction is thought to inhibit the target muscle neurologically and allow it to be stretched farther. Although reciprocal inhibition may not occur every time a muscle is activated, as described above, RI stretching can still be effective and references to "RI stretching" are still used by practitioners. Sport massage therapists often use RI stretching as a technique to relieve muscle cramps in athletes after strenuous effort. The therapist has the athlete isometrically contract the muscle opposite the cramping one, reciprocally inhibiting the cramping muscle, which then relaxes.

ACTIVE ISOLATED STRETCHING

Active isolated stretching (AIS) was developed by Aaron Mattes and is detailed in his book by the same name (Mattes 2000). This method uses active movement and RI, but not isometric work, to achieve greater flexibility. This type of stretching can also be performed with a partner as an active-assisted technique. Mattes recommends isolating the muscle to be stretched, then actively lengthening it to a point of "light irritation." He suggests holding this position for no more than 2 seconds, then returning the limb to the starting position. This sequence is usually repeated 8 to 10 times. This stretching protocol is thought to prevent the stretch reflex while activating RI, thereby allowing the target muscle to lengthen more easily.

PNF Stretching

Facilitated stretching is based on the principles of PNF and is one of several variations of PNF stretching. Other versions of PNF stretching are referred to as modified PNF (Moore and Hutton 1980; Cornelius and Craft-Hamm 1988), NF (Surburg 1981), and scientific stretching for sports (3-S technique; Holt 1976).

Most PNF stretching techniques are done passively or as active-assisted exercises. The two main types of PNF stretching, also called relaxation techniques by Voss and colleagues (1985), are hold-relax and contract-relax. These are described in more detail on pages 12-13.

Ballistic Stretching

Ballistic stretching is performed using rapid, bouncing movements to force the target muscle to elongate. This can be done actively or passively. Ballistic stretching is generally out of favor because it may elicit a strong myotatic stretch reflex and leave the muscle shorter than its prestretch length. Beaulieu (1981) asserts that ballistic stretching creates more than twice the tension in the target muscle that a static stretch does. This increases the likelihood of tearing the muscle, because the external force lengthening the muscle opposes the internal shortening force produced by the stretch reflex, resulting in excessive tension in the muscle and tendons (figure 1.5).

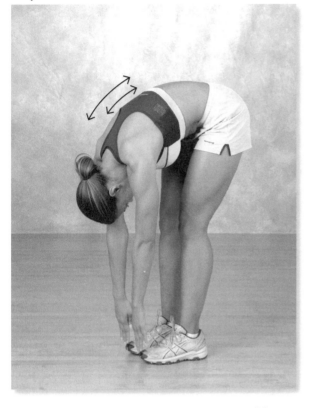

Figure 1.5 Ballistic stretching is performed using rapid, bouncing movements.

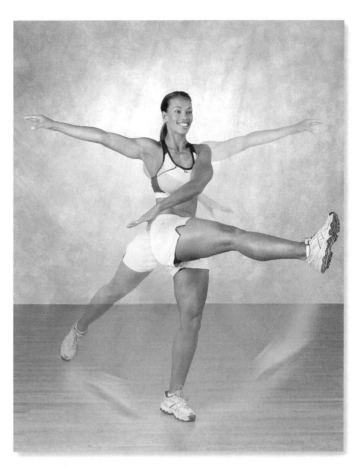

Figure 1.6 Dynamic stretching is characterized by controlled swings of a limb through its comfortable range of motion.

Dynamic Stretching

Dynamic flexibility refers to the ability to actively bring a limb through its full ROM. Dynamic stretching is usually performed as part of a warm-up prior to exercise and typically includes those muscles involved in the exercise or activity to be performed. Also called "dynamic range of motion" (DROM), dynamic stretching is achieved by moving a limb in a slow and controlled manner through its full available ROM. As the dynamic motion is repeated, the speed of the movement increases, as does the available ROM (Murphy 1994). Dynamic flexibility differs significantly from ballistic stretching because there are no bouncing or "jerky" movements, only controlled swings of the limb through its comfortable range (figure 1.6).

Static Stretching

Static stretching has been popularized by Bob Anderson in his book *Stretching* (2000). The muscle to be stretched (target muscle) is lengthened slowly (to inhibit firing of the stretch reflex) and held in a comfortable range for 15 to 30 seconds. As the position is held, the feeling of stretch diminishes and the stretcher moves gently into a deeper stretch and holds again. Static stretching can be done actively or passively (figure 1.7, *a* & *b*, p. 8).

Guidelines for Stretching

Despite years of research, there is still no clear agreement among the experts on whether stretching is worthwhile.

For years, the debate about stretching has been based on whether there are any tangible benefits. Proponents of stretching claim that it helps prevent injuries, prevents soreness, improves performance, promotes body awareness, stimulates blood flow, and is mentally relaxing and centering. Opponents argue that stretching is a waste of time, can actually cause injury, and does nothing to improve performance or

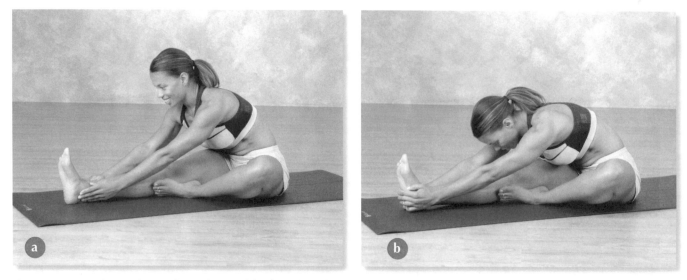

Figure 1.7 Hamstrings static stretch. *(a)* The stretch begins and *(b)* deepens after 15 to 30 seconds.

prevent soreness or injuries. Each side has a multitude of studies, reports, and anecdotal evidence to support its claims.

While we wait for the research to clearly elucidate the whole notion of stretching, we can find a consensus that favors stretching in conjunction with exercise. In the best of all possible exercise schemes, the athlete warms up, stretches, exercises, stretches again, and then cools down.

Stretch After Warm-Up

The physiological evidence is clear. When you stretch, it's more effective if the muscles are already warmed up. A warm-up entails 10 to 15 minutes of light activity, similar to what your exercise will be. This activity increases blood flow to the muscles you'll be using and gets them ready to work. Warming up also helps to reduce stiffness, making the muscles more supple, so they stretch more easily.

Grant (1997) discusses other benefits of warming up, including increased production of synovial fluid to lubricate joints, increased oxygen exchange in the muscle, increased rate of nerve transmission, and more efficient cooperation of the muscles around a joint. If you warm up first, your stretching exercises will be more effective and efficient, you'll make greater gains than if you're stretching cold, and you'll be less likely to injure yourself.

Stretch Twice

In an ideal world, we'd stretch after warming up, exercise, then stretch again after exercise as part of the cool-down process. The reasoning behind stretching twice goes like this:

1. Stretch the muscles before a workout to get them ready to perform at their optimum length. This optimum length allows the muscles to develop the most power as they work.

2. Stretch the muscles after exercise while they're still warm to bring them back to their optimum resting length. As muscles work they repeatedly contract and shorten, and they tend to stay short when the workout is over unless you stretch them again. Postexercise stretching can be incorporated into the cool-down.

Stretch Once

If time is limited, we recommend skipping the pre-exercise stretching and concentrating on postexercise stretching. If you don't stretch before exercise, be sure to complete a thorough warm-up before getting into your main workout. Postexercise stretching will return those tired muscles to their normal resting length as you go about the remainder of your daily activities. In postexercise stretching, there is some danger of overstretching the muscles because they may be too pliable. But if postexercise stretching is done with awareness, the risk is minimal and is far outweighed by the benefits.

Stretch Without Pain

Many people stretch incorrectly, believing that if something doesn't hurt a little, it's not working. We believe that stretching must be completely comfortable to be effective. If you stretch until it hurts, the body's natural response will be to tighten up to prevent any more lengthening, and possible injury, to the given muscle. We advocate stretching the muscle just to its "soft tissue barrier," that is, the point at which you begin to feel some resistance to further stretching but no discomfort. The soft tissue barrier is the starting point for the stretch.

Pain-free stretching also applies to the rest of the body during a specific stretch. If you are uncomfortable or in pain, even if you have no pain in the muscle you're stretching, your results will be less than optimal. For example, if you're having low back pain while you stretch your quadriceps, you won't be able to relax and fully engage in the stretch. Repositioning to relieve your back pain makes the quadriceps stretch more effective.

Remember That Flexibility Varies

Anyone who has been stretching for some time is acutely aware that flexibility varies from day to day and from joint to joint. Because of this, it's important to remember that stretching is not a contest. We take each day as it comes and stretch as best we can. Just as those who diet to lose weight are advised not to step on the scale daily, so too we can't measure improvement in flexibility daily, but are better off looking at our gains over the long term.

Recognize When to Stretch and When to Strengthen

Stretching tight muscles is a pleasurable activity when done correctly. But not all tight muscles need to be stretched. Some are already overstretched and need to be strengthened instead. The following paragraphs deal with the differences between hypertonic and eccentrically stressed muscles, "crossed syndrome," and the effects of neurological inhibition on muscle balance. This is a brief discussion of a complex topic, which we urge you to explore more fully in other writings devoted to the subject (Lewit (1999), Chaitow (2001), and Liebenson (1996)).

■ *Hypertonic muscles*—When a muscle is short and tight due to habitual concentric contraction, it's called hypertonic. Myers (2001) refers to this as "locked short." A good example of short and tight can be found in the pectoralis major. Because most of us spend so much time sitting in front of computers,

driving, or doing other activities that use our arms in front, the pectoralis muscles can become chronically hypertonic. Hypertonic muscles tend to feel fat or thick and tight to palpation. Stretching these muscles can help restore them to normal tone and length.

■ *Eccentrically stressed muscles*—When a muscle is overstretched (usually due to postural stress), it will also feel tight, but instead of being short and tight, it is long and tight, or "locked long" (Myers 2001). It stays in a state of eccentric contraction, in which it constantly works to try to return to its normal length. The rhomboids provide a good example of muscles under eccentric stress. Most of us tend to be a little round-shouldered. Hypertonic pectoralis muscles contribute to this posture. As a result, the rhomboids, which attach to the spine and the shoulder blades, are always fighting to counteract the force of the pectoralis muscles and pull the blades back to their normal position. The resulting eccentric stress causes the rhomboids to feel tight and sore to palpation. Muscles under eccentric stress tend to feel thin or stringy and tight. The correction for this condition is not to stretch the rhomboids, but to strengthen them and stretch the pectoralis muscles to restore balance between the chest and the back.

■ *Crossed syndrome*—Similar patterns of muscle imbalance can be found elsewhere in the body. Czech researcher Vladimir Janda (1983) describes these patterns of imbalance as upper and lower "crossed" syndromes.

■ *Muscle weakness due to inhibition*—Even though Sherrington's law of reciprocal inhibition does not universally apply as previously believed, our experience with patients has taught us to act as if hypertonic muscles have a reflexive inhibitory effect on their opposing muscles. To use the pectoralis muscles and the rhomboids again as an example, when the pectoralis muscles are locked short, they not only contribute to the eccentric stress on the rhomboids by mechanically pulling against them; they also appear to neurologically inhibit the rhomboids, making them less able to exert their normal strength to maintain postural balance. It is common to find that the rhomboids regain much of their normal strength and tone spontaneously after the pectoralis muscles are released through stretching. The same scenario is seen in many areas of the body. Because of this, we believe that stretching work should precede strengthening when one is trying to correct postural imbalances.

Focusing on Facilitated Stretching

Most of us know that stretching is an important part of training for any sport. Beyond sport, stretching is useful for maintaining general flexibility for daily activities and as preventive maintenance in repetitive motion activities. As we saw in chapter 1, there are many ways to stretch, from the overall stretches we do naturally to specific techniques found in the many books available today. Facilitated stretching is an active-assisted stretching technique based on the theories and principles of proprioceptive neuromuscular facilitation (PNF), a physical therapy modality.

Overview of PNF

Before moving on to facilitated stretching, we'll begin by discussing the history of PNF and reviewing its spiral–diagonal movement patterns.

Brief History of PNF

PNF is a treatment technique that was developed in the mid-twentieth century by Herman Kabat, MD, PhD, and two physical therapists, Margaret "Maggie" Knott and Dorothy Voss. Kabat, a neurophysiologist, based much of the theoretical structure of PNF on the work of Sir Charles Sherrington, whose research in the early to mid-1900s helped develop a model for how the neuromuscular system operates (Sherrington 1947).

Dr. Kabat believed that the principles of neurophysiological development and Sherrington's laws of irradiation, successive induction, and reciprocal innervation should be applied in the rehabilitation of polio patients with paralysis. Before the development of PNF techniques, paralyzed patients had been rehabilitated using methods that emphasized "one motion, one joint, one muscle at a time" (Voss, Ionta, and Myers 1985).

With backing from industrialist Henry Kaiser, Dr. Kabat founded the Kabat-Kaiser Institute (KKI) in Washington, DC, in 1946 and began working with paralysis patients to find combinations and patterns of movement that were consistent with neurophysiological theory. By 1951, Kabat and Knott had identified and established nine techniques for rehabilitating muscles.

Physical therapist Dorothy Voss became interested in PNF in 1950 as she learned from and worked with Knott. She was hired as Knott's assistant in 1952. Voss and Knott realized that PNF was more than a system for the treatment of paralysis; it was a new way of thinking about and using movement and therapeutic exercise.

In 1952 Knott and Voss began presenting workshops to train other physical therapists in PNF methods. By 1954 they were conducting two-week training programs, and in 1956 they published the first edition of *Proprioceptive Neuromuscular Facilitation*.

During the 1960s, PNF courses became available through physical therapy departments at several universities, and their popularity continued to grow. Now PNF techniques are taught as undergraduate course work in most physical therapy programs.

Over the past 20 years, PNF stretching methods have gained popularity, especially in the athletic community and increasingly with the general public. PNF stretching is only one component of the entire PNF repertoire. PNF stretching uses an isometric contraction prior to the stretch to achieve greater gains than those that would be achieved with stretching alone. PNF stretching is generally done passively; that is, the physical therapist does the stretching for the patient.

Basis of PNF: Spiral–Diagonal Movement

PNF is based on spiral–diagonal movement. Kabat and Knott observed that normal movements seen in sports and physical activities are spiral–diagonal in nature. They defined these "mass movement patterns" as "various combinations of motion . . . [that] require shortening and lengthening reactions of many muscles in varying degrees" (Voss, Ionta, and Myers 1985). The spiral–diagonal character of normal movements arises from the design of the skeletal system and the placement of the muscles on it. The muscles spiral around the bones from origin to insertion, and therefore, when they contract, they tend to create that spiral in motion. The motions required when you comb your hair, swing a golf club, or kick a ball all have spiral (rotational) and diagonal components; that is, they occur not in straight lines, but through several planes of motion. If you look at figure 2.1, you can see that the bowler's right arm is moving not only forward, but also diagonally up and across his body. You'll also see the spiral component of his motion if you look at the rotation of his arm. Spiral–diagonal motion is also taking place at his left arm and left leg (figure 2.1).

From PNF Stretching to Facilitated Stretching

As we mentioned in chapter 1, facilitated stretching is one of several variations of PNF stretching.

Most PNF stretching techniques are done passively or as active-assisted exercises. The two main

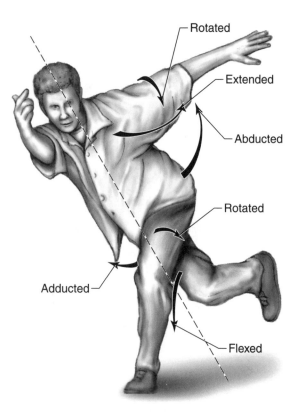

Figure 2.1 The bowler illustrates arm movement with three components of motion: forward, diagonally across, and rotating. Spiral–diagonal motion is also occurring at his left arm and left leg.

types, also called relaxation techniques by Voss and colleagues (1985), are hold-relax and contract-relax.

PNF Hold-Relax

Hold-relax (HR) is generally used if range of motion is extremely limited or if active movement is not available because of weakness or pain.

The stretcher holds the limb at its lengthened range of motion and isometrically resists the therapist's attempt to move the limb into a deeper stretch of the target muscle. The stretcher then relaxes and actively moves the limb into the new range (figure 2.2).

PNF Contract-Relax

Contract-relax (CR) is used with patients who exhibit a marked limitation in range of motion. This technique combines isotonic and isometric work in the spiral patterns of PNF. Using CR, the physical therapist moves the limb passively to the point of limitation,

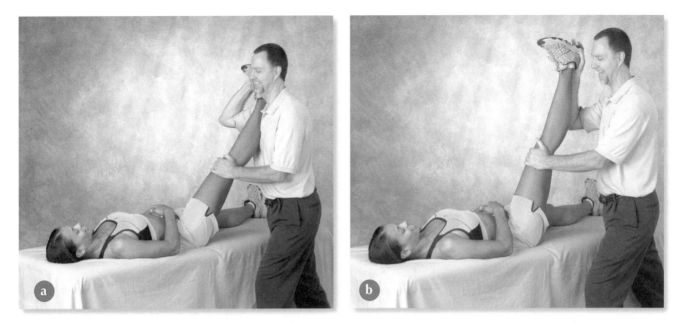

Figure 2.2   The PNF hold-relax stretch for the hamstrings. *(a)* The stretcher isometrically contracts her hamstrings to resist the partner's attempt to move her leg farther into flexion. *(b)* The stretcher actively moves into a deeper stretch.

then instructs the patient to try to move the limb into the shortened range. The physical therapist resists but allows rotation of the limb, an isotonic contraction. All other directional effort by the patient is isometric. After the contraction, the therapist moves the limb passively into a new range of motion. After several rounds of CR, the patient is instructed to move actively through the new range of motion.

With facilitated stretching we rely on the principles and techniques of PNF, including the use of isometric contractions, the isolation of muscles through proper positioning, and the use of the spiral–diagonal pattern. With facilitated stretching, the emphasis is on active, rather than passive, stretching, meaning that the stretcher does most or all of the work. When a partner is involved, the partner's job is to monitor and direct the stretcher's activity.

Facilitated stretching can bring about dramatic gains in flexibility in a very short time because the protocol we use facilitates a muscle's ability to lengthen.

Guidelines for Performing Facilitated Stretches

Although facilitated stretching is an easy technique to learn, there are important, if subtle, factors to understand. In this section, we describe an easy-to-

remember three-step stretching protocol, then discuss critical elements of the technique that must be applied to achieve optimum results.

Follow This Three-Step Sequence

Facilitated stretching is active-assisted stretching, using active motion and isometric work to improve flexibility and enhance motor learning in the process. Simplified, the three steps involved in facilitated stretching are:

1. The stretcher actively lengthens the muscle to be stretched (target muscle).
2. The stretcher isometrically contracts the target muscle for 6 seconds.
3. The stretcher actively stretches the target muscle to a new range of motion.

For example, to stretch the hamstrings, the stretcher begins by contracting the quadriceps and psoas (hip flexors) to actively move his leg to the starting position, without assistance. She then isometrically contracts his hamstrings for 6 seconds as the partner provides resistance. Finally, by contracting the hip flexors again to lift the leg higher, the stretcher actively stretches the hamstrings to a new length (figure 2.3, a-c, p. 14).

The three-step sequence of facilitated stretching has developed over years of clinical practice. It was

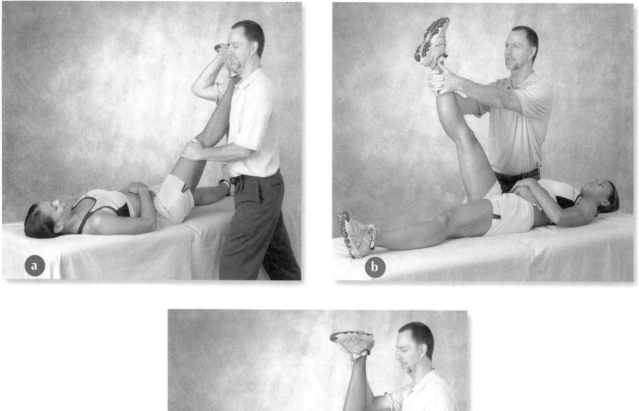

Figure 2.3 Facilitated stretch for the hamstrings. *(a)* Starting position of the hamstrings stretch (right leg). Support the leg using proper biomechanics. The partner offers resistance only to match the stretcher's isometric contraction of the hamstrings. *(b)* This photo illustrates an alternate position for the partner. *(c)* The stretcher actively moves into a deeper stretch with no help from the partner.

originally based on the premise that we were activating two neurological effects: reciprocal inhibition and postisometric relaxation. As we discussed in chapter 1, current scientific consensus is that these effects may not consistently occur as previously believed. Unfortunately, we have no firm evidence of the physiological reasons that stretching is so much more effective using facilitated techniques. Research points to two promising hypotheses: an "increased tolerance to stretch" or changes in the viscoelastic properties of the stretched muscle (Chalmers 2002, 2004).

Empower the Stretcher to Take an Active Role

In addition to its effectiveness, there is a deeper, philosophical basis for using facilitated stretching over other styles. Passive forms of stretching, in which the partner does the stretching to or for the stretcher, encourage the stretcher to become dependent on a partner. Facilitated stretching is active; and because the stretcher gains flexibility easily using these techniques, she will be more motivated to continue stretching on her own. This helps avoid making the stretcher dependent on someone else and encourages her own body awareness. With facilitated stretching, the stretcher learns to do the work for herself and becomes more body aware in the process.

One of the challenges with any stretching technique is maintaining consistent practice. Facilitated stretching is done by the stretcher, and the partner acts only as a facilitator. Self-stretching is emphasized so that the stretcher can do it alone, using a stretching strap, a doorway, or a piece of exercise equipment at the gym to replace the partner. These self-stretching techniques are easy to learn. Also, because the stretcher is motivated when he sees results, and because the techniques engage the mind and the body, he will be much more likely to continue practicing the stretches as part of a home program.

Engage Muscles to Improve Neuromuscular Function

Facilitated stretching is designed to improve the communication between the muscles and the nervous system. The muscles do only what they are told to do by the nervous system. Therefore, this interaction must be clear. When the muscles are actively engaged throughout the routine, learning takes place that allows them to work more efficiently. In passive stretching, this does not occur because the outside force is doing most of the work, with little neurological or muscular involvement required of the stretcher.

Use Action Verbs

In general, during the isometric phase your instruction to the stretcher will be an action verb like "push," "pull," "turn," "twist," or "kick." This communicates clearly what you wish to have happen. If you ask the stretcher to "resist," you are communicating that you will be doing something to her that she needs to act against. In fact, you want her to contract the muscle, whose force you, as the facilitator, will resist. The use of action verbs also relates to our discussion of empowering the stretcher to take an active, rather than passive, role in the process.

Encourage Normal Breathing

Muscles need oxygen to work. But we are often in the habit of holding our breath during strong muscular effort. How do we reconcile these two conflicting facts? We think it's more important to breathe, especially because we are not asking for maximal effort on the part of the stretcher during any part of the sequence. Secondly, holding the breath during the

isometric phase is often accompanied by compensatory recruitment of other muscles. And third, there is some risk that holding the breath during muscular contraction may raise the blood pressure.

It's easy to monitor the stretcher's breathing and your own throughout the process. We've found that two to three cycles of normal breathing (in and out) takes about 6 seconds, which is the length of time we want for the isometric contraction.

Recognize the Importance of Positioning

To achieve the greatest benefit from stretching, the goal is to position the stretcher to isolate the target muscle as much as possible. This isolation ensures that the target muscle is the primary one contracting during the isometric phase and being stretched during the lengthening phase. Although it's impossible to completely isolate and activate only one muscle,

Self-Stretching Principles

In keeping with the theme of stretcher learning and self-help, our goal is to teach the stretcher to incorporate facilitated stretching into his daily routine without the need to rely on a partner. During partner stretching sessions, the partner can point out compensation patterns, emphasize different aspects of a particular spiral pattern, and fine-tune the technique. In a home program, the learning is reinforced through daily practice, and the stretcher's overall flexibility or rehabilitation (or both) progresses more quickly. For these reasons, most of the stretches presented here include a self-stretch version. The principles for self-stretching are identical to the ones for partner work:

- Use proper positioning to isolate the target muscle.
- Use self-stabilization to prevent compensation.
- Breathe correctly.
- Exert appropriate effort during the isometric phase.
- Stretch the target muscle by contracting the opposing muscle.
- Remain pain free throughout the sequence.

careless positioning allows inappropriate muscle recruitment and interferes with achieving optimum results from facilitated stretching.

Because the stretcher does most of the work in facilitated stretching, it's common to see compensation patterns occurring, especially during the isometric phase. For this reason, we need to pay attention to the stretcher's mechanics and stabilization.

Be Aware of Compensation Patterns

We all develop compensatory patterns of muscular contraction to make up for muscle weakness or imbalance, postural distortions, structural irregularities, and the like. When we are performing facilitated stretching, many of these patterns of compensation become obvious. For instance, in facilitating a hamstrings stretch, we very often see the hip lift off the table when the stretcher is isometrically contracting the hamstrings. This unconscious shift engages the gluteus maximus more and is usually the result of a weak hamstring.

By being aware of compensation and working with the stretcher to eliminate it during facilitated stretching, we'll achieve better results on the table, and the stretcher will learn to move more efficiently as she goes about her daily life. Where appropriate, we've indicated the common compensation patterns associated with a stretch.

It's valuable for the stretcher to take an active role in preventing compensation during the stretching work. This active learning translates into her daily life. If the stretcher can learn to use her gluteus maximus and hamstrings without compensation on the table, then she'll be more likely to carry that new, correct behavior into her everyday activities.

There's another component of greater involvement on the part of the stretcher in stabilizing her motion: the discovery of aspects she has been unaware of. For example, in attempting to stretch the quadratus lumborum, many people are unable to isolate the muscle. They begin recruiting like mad to try to do the simple motion required for the stretch. This discovery enables us to work together to figure out how to simply contract the quadratus lumborum without engaging other muscles inappropriately. The learning that results is extremely useful for the stretcher as she incorporates it into her daily life.

Detailed Sequence for Facilitated Stretching

As mentioned earlier, facilitated stretching is usually done with a partner, although many of the stretches can be done alone, assisted by accessories. The more detailed steps involved in a partner-assisted facilitated stretch are as follows:

1. The stretcher actively lengthens the muscle to be stretched (the target muscle) to its maximal pain-free end range. This is also called the soft tissue barrier or stretch barrier.

   For example, if you wish to stretch the hamstrings, have the stretcher lie on her back and contract her quadriceps and psoas (hip flexors) to actively lift the leg as high as possible, keeping the knee straight. You may need to hold the knee straight as the stretcher lifts her leg. This stretches the hamstrings to their end range (figure 2.3a, p. 14).

2. As the partner, position yourself to offer resistance for the stretcher to isometrically contract the target muscle against. For stretching the hamstrings, support the lower leg against your shoulder or by holding it with both hands (figure 2.3b).

3. Direct the stretcher to begin slowly and "push" or "pull" to isometrically contract the target muscle as you provide matching resistance. Don't allow the stretcher to overpower you. When the stretcher has achieved the proper level of isometric contraction (strong, but not maximum strength), hold it for 6 seconds.

4. After the 6-second contraction, the stretcher relaxes and inhales deeply. During this time, maintain the limb in the starting position.

5. As she exhales, the stretcher contracts the opposing muscles, in this case the quads and psoas, and pulls the target muscle into a deeper stretch (figure 2.3c). As the partner, do not push or pull to force the stretch.

6. Now, as the partner, you will move into the new position to once again offer resistance.

7. Repeat the process two to three times.

Facilitated stretches should always be pain free. If the stretcher experiences pain, try repositioning the limb or use less force during the isometric contraction of the target muscle. If pain persists, don't use the technique for that particular muscle until you've determined why it's causing pain.

Safety Considerations for Facilitated Stretching

Facilitated stretches, also known as CRAC stretches (contract, relax, agonist contract), entail virtually no risk of injury because there is little or no passive movement involved—the stretcher does the work. You act only as a facilitator for the technique and make no attempt to increase the stretch. This factor addresses the concern of some investigators that poorly trained or inattentive partners could cause injury by being too vigorous in moving the limb to a new range of motion (Beaulieu 1981; Surburg 1981).

Stretching safely is of utmost concern for both the stretcher and the partner. Using proper body mechanics is extremely important during all phases of stretching, but especially during the isometric phase. The stretcher and the partner need to plan carefully and communicate freely with each other. The partner may be expending unnecessary energy (because of poor ergonomics) in applying the resistance, or the stretcher may be working too hard. As the partner you can be injured by carelessly using these techniques and you can develop overuse syndromes unnecessarily.

Safety for the Partner

When you are acting as the partner during facilitated stretching, you may be at risk for injury if you don't take care of yourself. By paying attention to your posture and body mechanics, you can eliminate the possibility of injury. Remember these points:

▪ As you work, pay attention to your legs and feet. Use an "athletic stance" to help you remain balanced and stable, especially as you resist the isometric contraction of the stretcher. This stance will usually be a variation on a lunge, with one foot forward and the other back. The legs are set wide apart; the knees are usually slightly bent; the back is relatively straight; the head is upright; body weight is evenly distributed; and the use of the powerful leg muscles is stressed (figure 2.4).

▪ Be aware of keeping your spine lengthened as you work, instead of collapsing into yourself. This lengthening helps prevent undue stress on your vertebrae.

▪ Keep your low back area flattened to reduce pressure on your lumbar spine. This will help prevent low back pain. Tighten your abdominal muscles to help keep your back from arching too far.

▪ Avoid unnecessary twisting or bending. Instead, have the stretcher move to accommodate you.

▪ Use the large muscles of the trunk and extremities to resist the isometric contraction instead of smaller, weaker muscles. For instance, have the stretcher push against your shoulder rather than your arm during a hamstrings stretch.

▪ Remember that you control the strength of the stretcher's isometric contraction. Provide resistance

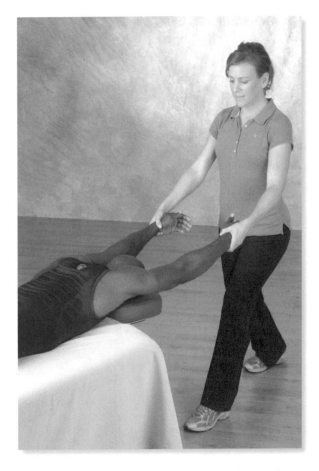

Figure 2.4 This photo illustrates a version of the "athletic stance," a modified lunge with the pelvis turned toward the line of force.

only up to the level that is comfortable for you; then ask the stretcher to hold at that level of effort. It is not necessary for the stretcher to exert maximal effort for the technique to work.

▪ To avoid losing your balance when you're acting as the partner, you need to control the session and give the commands so that you're prepared to resist the isometric contraction. Be sure that the stretcher begins slowly during the isometric phase.

▪ Stop immediately if either you or the stretcher has pain, discuss what is happening to determine the cause, and correct the problem before continuing.

Safety for the Stretcher

When a stretcher is first learning facilitated stretching, it is common for him to work too hard, to lose focus, and to misunderstand the directions for each stretch. To keep the stretcher safe, be sure to proceed slowly, make sure he understands your instructions, and prevent him from overworking.

It's important to be sure that the stretcher is positioned correctly for the stretch, that he is breathing throughout the sequence, and that he is pain free throughout.

Reducing Fatigue for Stretcher and Partner

Because facilitated stretching is an active form of work, it can be fatiguing for both the stretcher and the partner. Preventing fatigue can reduce the chance of injury.

For the stretcher, it's important to remember that maximal effort is not necessary. We need only a moderate contraction of the target muscle during the isometric phase. This can be especially important for stretchers who don't participate in a regular exercise program, because they may experience muscle soreness the next day if they work too hard.

For you, the partner, reducing fatigue becomes an issue if you are working with several people throughout the day. Injuries are more likely if you're fatigued. One of the benefits of facilitated stretching is that the stretcher does most of the work. As the partner, your main task is to assist the stretcher, not do the work for her. The stretcher moves the limb into position; you don't have to lift it or support it for her except for brief periods during the sequence. Relax whenever possible during the session and expend only the effort necessary.

If you're using proper body mechanics, you will usually have a mechanical advantage when resisting the isometric contraction of the stretcher. This leverage allows you to accomplish your work with minimal physical effort.

CHAPTER 3

Using the Spiral-Diagonal Patterns of PNF

You recall that PNF is based on spiral–diagonal patterns of movement. This spiral–diagonal nature of normal movements arises from the design of the skeletal system and the placement of the muscles on it. The muscles spiral around the bones from origin to insertion, and therefore, when they contract, they tend to create that spiral in motion.

This spiral is especially noticeable in the movements of your arms, which swing across your body as you walk or run. When the biceps contract, they not only flex your elbow but also rotate (supinate) your forearm. Many muscles are actually capable of motion in three planes (figure 3.1, *a-d,* p. 20). For instance, the psoas muscle flexes the hip (the dominant action) but also assists adduction and external rotation of the femur (figure 3.2, p. 21).

Movement that is devoid of spiral and diagonal motion looks and feels stiff, awkward, and clumsy. Coordinated, graceful movement can be compromised through outright injury, or more insidiously when we limit our movement patterns through habituation. One of the primary benefits of learning and using the spiral patterns of PNF is to restore or enhance coordinated, graceful movement that incorporates multiple planes and axes of motion.

Practicing the Patterns as Free Movement

Voss and colleagues (1985) suggest learning the spiral patterns through free-movement exercises. These give a sense of the natural rhythm of the patterns and let you feel the movements through a full range of motion. Even though we don't use the full patterns in facilitated stretching, learning them will make it easier to visualize the range of motion you're trying to improve as you incorporate these patterns into stretching.

These patterns can be used to help improve your own coordination and can be made more challenging when you move both arms simultaneously, completing a different pattern with each arm, or add a leg pattern into the mix. Try it and have some fun as you explore the connections between your brain and your muscles.

Patterns for the Arm

There are two basic PNF patterns for the arm: Diagonal one (D1) and Diagonal two (D2). Each pattern can be divided into two parts: flexion and extension. The movement sequence for the D1 extension pattern is

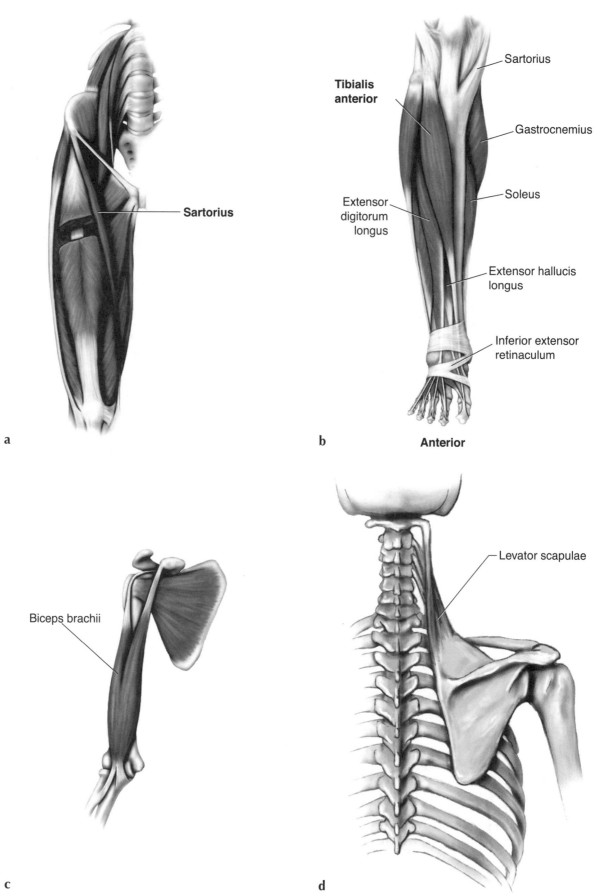

Sartorius

a

Tibialis anterior

Sartorius

Gastrocnemius

Soleus

Extensor digitorum longus

Extensor hallucis longus

Inferior extensor retinaculum

b   **Anterior**

Biceps brachii

c

Levator scapulae

d

Figure 3.1 The attachments of the *(a)* sartorius, *(b)* tibialis anterior, *(c)* biceps brachii, and *(d)* levator scapulae muscles facilitate spiral–diagonal motion when the muscles contract.

Nomenclature Change From Previous Editions

In previous editions of *Facilitated Stretching*, we adhered to the nomenclature for PNF used in physical therapy, naming the patterns based on their ending position. For instance, if I start at the flexion end of D1 (flexion, adduction, and external rotation), the motion goes in the opposite direction, ending at the extension end of D1 (extension, abduction, and internal rotation). We have called this D1 Extension. This has produced some confusion, because in using the patterns for stretching, we never actually complete the motion to the opposite direction but only attempt it isometrically. In practice, we usually talk about stretching into the flexion end or the extension end of D1 or D2. So, in this edition, we have abandoned the earlier method of naming and have gone with the simplified and more accurate description that we use in practice.

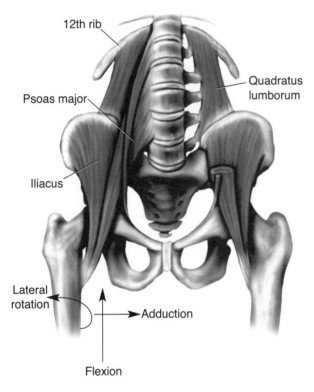

Figure 3.2   **The iliopsoas, like many muscles, is capable of producing motion through three planes of movement.**

the exact opposite of the sequence for D1 flexion. The same is true for D2 extension and D2 flexion.

D1 PATTERN FOR THE ARM

Diagonal one (D1) can be divided into D1 flexion and D1 extension. D1 flexion finishes with the arm in flexion, adduction, and external rotation, which means it begins in the opposite position of extension, abduction, and internal rotation. D1 extension finishes with the arm in extension, abduction, and internal rotation, so must begin in flexion, adduction, and external rotation (see figure 3.3, p. 22).

This makes more sense when you perform the pattern instead of just reading about it. So take a moment now and practice D1 before going on.

D1 Practice: Arm

1. Stand and bring your right arm up and across your body, with your arm rotated so that the thumb side of your hand points forward, as in figure 3.3*a*. Specifically, this is flexion, horizontal adduction, and external rotation of the humerus. The right forearm is supinated, and the wrist and fingers are flexed.

2. Go as far in each plane of motion as you can to fully lengthen all the involved muscles. This is the ending position for D1 flexion.

3. From this starting position, slowly rotate and move your arm diagonally, down, out, and back to arrive at the same arm and hand position as shown in figure 3.3*b*. This motion blends internal rotation, abduction, and extension of the humerus, pronation of the forearm, and extension of the wrist and fingers. This is the ending position for D1 extension.

4. From this position, retrace your motion to arrive once again at the flexion end of D1.

Repetition, Repetition

Repeat these patterns several times with each arm, and then with both together, until you feel the rhythm. What activities use motion like this? Throwing a Frisbee, swinging a golf club or a baseball bat, picking up a hat and putting it on your head, working as a grocery checker, feeding yourself, and using a seat belt in your car all use patterns of movement that have components of the D1 pattern. It may help you remember the ends of the two patterns by giving them nicknames. Think of D1 flexion, figure 3.3*a*, as the "grab seat belt" pattern. "Fasten seat belt," as in figure 3.3*b*, puts you in D1 extension.

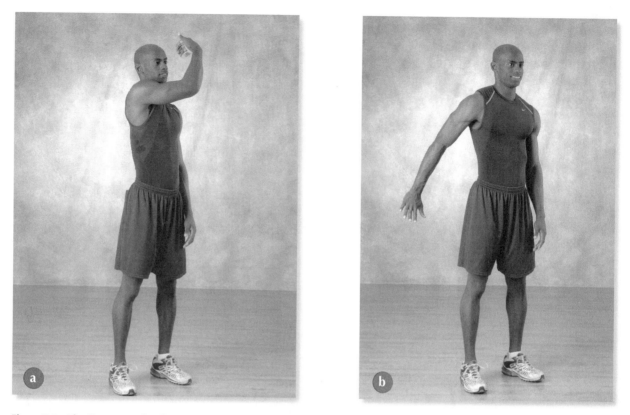

Figure 3.3 The D1 pattern for the arm. *(a)* The flexion end of D1 ("grab seat belt"), and *(b)* the extension end of D1 ("fasten seat belt").

D2 PATTERN FOR THE ARM

Diagonal two (D2) uses the diagonal line opposite to that for D1 and is divided into D2 flexion and D2 extension. D2 flexion finishes with the arm in flexion, abduction, and external rotation. D2 extension finishes with the arm in extension, adduction, and internal rotation (see figure 3.4).

Once again, the patterns make more sense when you perform them. So take some time to practice D2 now, before going on.

D2 Practice: Arm

1. Stand and bring your right arm up, out, and slightly behind your body, with your arm rotated so the thumb faces behind you, as in figure 3.4a. This is flexion, abduction, and external rotation of the humerus. The right forearm is supinated, with the wrist and fingers extended.

2. Go as far in each plane of motion as you can to fully lengthen all the involved muscles. This is the ending position for D2 flexion.

3. From this starting position, slowly rotate and move your arm diagonally down and across your body, as if you were putting a sword back

into its scabbard, ending up in the same position as the model in figure 3.4b. This motion blends internal rotation, adduction, and extension of the humerus. The forearm pronates, and the wrist and fingers flex. For the sake of practice, you are now at the ending position for D2 extension. In reality, the ending position would be through the body, in a "hammerlock" position, to ensure that the arm is fully extended and internally rotated.

4. Now, retrace your motion to arrive back at the flexion end of D2.

Repetition, Repetition

Repeat these patterns several times with each arm, and then with both together, until they begin to feel natural and easy. What activities use motion like this? Throwing a ball, drawing a sword, using a hockey stick, lifting and stacking, washing windows, and taking a sweater off over your head all use patterns of movement that have components of the D2 pattern. Again, it may help you remember the ends of the patterns by giving them nicknames. We'll call D2 flexion (figure 3.4a) "drawing a sword" and D2 extension (figure 3.4b) "sheathing a sword."

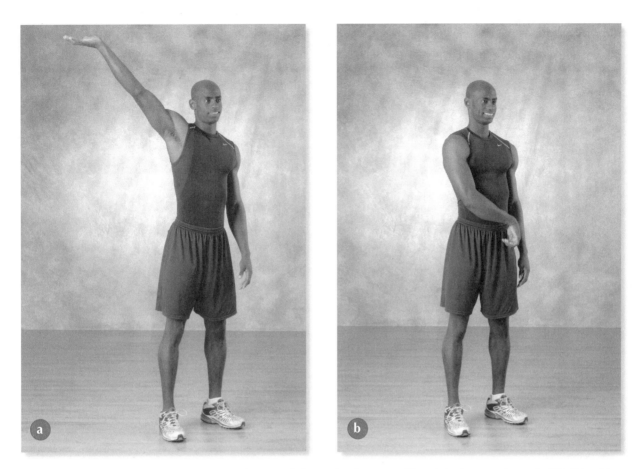

Figure 3.4 The D2 pattern for the arm. *(a)* The flexion end of D2 ("drawing a sword"), and *(b)* the extension end of D2 ("sheathing a sword").

Patterns for the Leg

When you feel competent with the arm patterns, you can move on to the legs. As with the arm, there are two patterns for the leg: D1 and D2. These can also be divided into two parts: flexion and extension. The leg patterns are similar to those for the arms, but not identical.

D1 PATTERN FOR THE LEG

Diagonal one (D1) can be divided into D1 flexion and D1 extension. D1 flexion finishes with the leg in flexion, adduction, and external rotation. D1 extension finishes with the leg in extension, abduction, and internal rotation (see figure 3.5, p. 24).

Active practice will make this easier to understand. You'll find it easier to do this practice if you hold onto something for balance and support.

D1 Practice: Leg

1. Stand and bring your right leg forward and across your body, rotating the leg so your foot points to the right. This is flexion, adduction, and external

rotation of the femur, dorsiflexion and inversion of the foot, and extension of the toes.

2. Go as far in each plane of motion as you can to fully lengthen all the involved muscles. This is the ending position for D1 flexion. Check your position against that shown in figure 3.5a.

3. Slowly swing the leg, beginning with internal rotation, to end up with the leg behind and away from your body, with the foot pointing to the left. This is extension, abduction, and internal rotation of the femur, plantarflexion and eversion of the foot, and flexion of the toes. Compare your position with that of the model in figure 3.5b. This is the ending position for D1 extension.

4. From this position, retrace your motion to return to the flexion end of D1.

Repetition, Repetition

Swing your leg through this pattern several times to feel the rhythm of it. Many athletic activities require aspects of the D1 pattern. Dancers, skaters, and

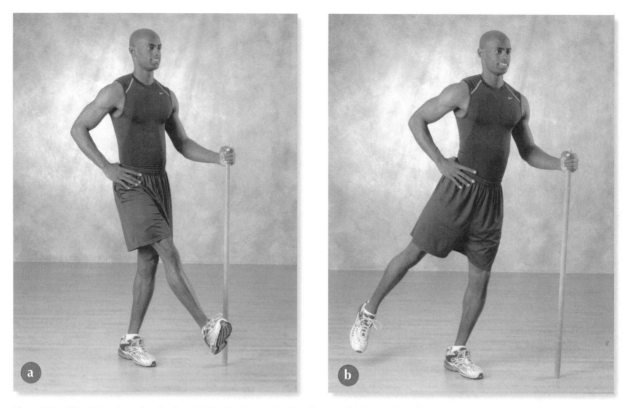

Figure 3.5   **The D1 pattern for the leg.** *(a)* **The flexion end of D1 ("soccer kick") and** *(b)* **the extension end of D1 ("toe-off").**

soccer players, to name a few, all need coordination and flexibility through the D1 pattern. D1 flexion (figure 3.5*a*) is called the "soccer kick." You can remember D1 extension (figure 3.5*b*) as "toe-off."

D2 PATTERN FOR THE LEG

Diagonal two (D2) uses the diagonal line opposite to D1 and is also divided into D2 flexion and D2 extension. D2 flexion ends in flexion, abduction, and internal rotation of the leg. D2 extension ends in extension, adduction, and external rotation (see figure 3.6).

Active practice makes it clearer.

D2 Practice: Leg

1. Stand and bring your right leg forward and out away from your body, rotating the leg so your foot points to the left. This is flexion, abduction, and internal rotation. The foot is dorsiflexed and everted, and the toes are extended.

2. Go as far in each plane of motion as you can to fully lengthen all the involved muscles. This is the ending position for D2 flexion. Compare your position to that of the model in figure 3.6*a*.

3. Slowly swing your leg behind and across your body, rotating the leg externally. This is exten-

sion, adduction, and external rotation of the femur. The foot is plantarflexed and inverted, and the toes are flexed.

4. Go as far in each plane of motion as you can to fully lengthen all the involved muscles. You've achieved the end of D2 extension. Check your position with that shown in figure 3.6*b*.

Repetition, Repetition

As you practice this D2 pattern a few times, does it remind you of any activity? If you're a skier, you may recognize components of the snowplow turn in D2 flexion. To help you remember it, we'll call D2 flexion (figure 3.6*a*) the "snowplow." D2 extension reminds some people of a ballet position, so we'll call D2 extension (figure 3.6*b*) "5th position."

Stretching With the Patterns

The full spiral–diagonal patterns move through three planes of motion: extension or flexion, adduction or abduction, and internal or external rotation. When the goal is to restore or increase strength and coordination, as well as to increase range of motion, moving through the whole diagonal pattern is the most effective strategy.

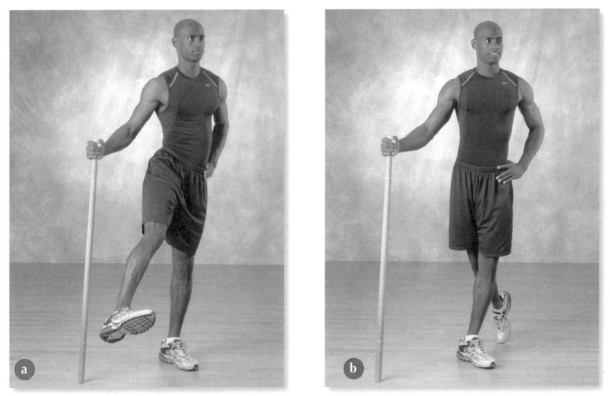

Figure 3.6   The D2 pattern for the leg. (a) The flexion end of D2 ("snowplow"), and (b) the extension end of D2 ("5th position").

Work at the End of Range

In facilitated stretching, our primary goal is to increase range of motion quickly and effectively, rather than improving strength and coordination.

For this reason, we employ only the lengthened position of the pattern, preventing the limb from going through its full range of motion. The stretcher assumes the ending position of the pattern (lengthened range), but her attempts to move the limb to the opposite end of the pattern are isometric; that is, she pushes or pulls in all three planes of motion, but no movement occurs. The stretch occurs after the isometric phase, when the stretcher actively moves farther into the lengthened range of the pattern.

Blend Adduction and Flexion or Abduction and Extension

When we're using the patterns, our goal is to emphasize the diagonal line of stretch. For instance, in the flexion end of the D1 pattern, we don't want too much adduction, or too much flexion, but a blend of the two. It may be helpful to visualize a diagonal line through opposite corners of the table or the stretching mat on which the stretcher is lying. You can use this diagonal line as a guide for the move-

ment of the arm or leg to be sure you have a balanced blend of adduction and flexion or abduction and extension (figure 3.7).

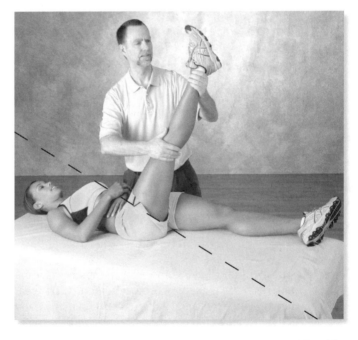

Figure 3.7   Visualize a diagonal line through opposite corners of the table. Use this line as a guide for the movement of the leg to be sure you have a balanced blend of flexion and adduction.

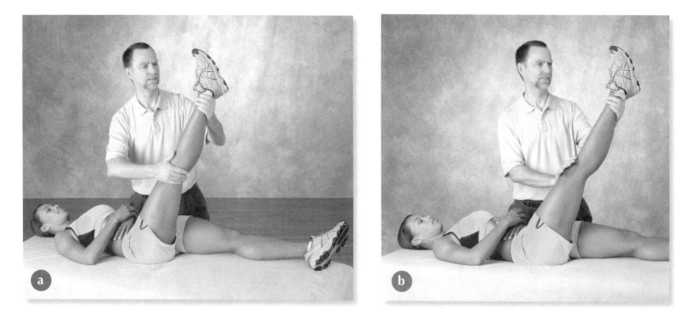

Figure 3.8 Hand contacts as the stretcher is asked to push "down and out." *(a)* Correct hand placement and *(b)* incorrect hand placement.

Although this blend of motion is usually what we're looking for, there may be times when you wish to emphasize one over the other. For instance, you may find that the stretcher's motion is more limited in adduction than in flexion. You can improve her range in adduction by deviating from the diagonal to emphasize more adduction and less flexion.

Maintain Precise Hand Contacts

Physical therapists emphasize the importance of precise hand contacts in PNF. Neurologically, the client wants to push or pull against the contact.

When you place your hands on the medial side of the limb, you should be verbally directing the stretcher to push or pull in that direction. Asking for a lateral push while holding on the medial side may be very confusing to the stretcher because your verbal commands don't match the proprioceptive cues your hands are communicating (figure 3.8).

Strengthening With the Patterns

We have found that incorporating the spiral–diagonal patterns into an exercise program can provide great benefit. Since the spiral patterns occur in many daily activities, as well as in sports, using the patterns to consciously improve strength, endurance, and coordination throughout these movements is a natural progression from the stretching work.

There are many ways to use the patterns in training, whether at the gym, on the road, or in a home program. We particularly like using stability balls and elastic bands. In the gym, wall-mounted pulley systems are easily adaptable to pattern work. Some of the newer free-standing gym equipment is also well suited to training in the spiral patterns.

In these next few pages, we provide you with some general ideas and suggestions for strengthening exercises that are performed with elastic bands. We recommend that you consult a certified personal trainer or strength coach to help design the program appropriate for you.

Surgical tubing or elastic bands are generally available through medical supply houses, physical therapy clinics, and stores or catalogs devoted to exercise and fitness equipment. Bands and tubing are usually color coded to indicate the level of resistance they provide. Deciding on the resistance level that's right for you is somewhat a matter of trial and error, but generally, starting with a midlevel band will work for most readers. You can adjust the amount of work you do by changing the length of the band as you exercise.

Instructions are written for the right arm or leg. Be sure to repeat all exercises on the left.

Strengthening the Arms

Once you have become sufficiently familiar with the spiral patterns for the arms by practicing them as general warm-ups, you can begin to focus on using them for a strength workout. Don't work too hard at the beginning of your program, because you may find that you're too sore the next day. It's best to start slowly and work your way up to a more strenuous routine.

D1 FLEXION: ARMS

To improve the strength, endurance, and coordination of the muscles in this pattern (front of the chest and shoulder), attach one end of the elastic band to a fixed object behind you at floor level. Hold the other end of the band in your right hand and place your arm in extension, abduction, and internal rotation ("fasten seat belt"). Take up the slack on the band by wrapping it around your hand or by stepping a little farther away from it (figure 3.9, *a-b*, p. 28).

From this starting position, begin a slow and controlled motion to reach up and across your body toward your left shoulder, ending at the flexion end of D1 (flexion, adduction, external rotation: "grab seat belt"). Your goal is to complete this spiral motion with ease and grace! If you can't, adjust your starting position to reduce the resistance on the band.

Once you've reached the end of D1 flexion, begin a slow and controlled return to your starting position. You may find this eccentric contraction (or negative work) more difficult.

That makes one repetition. Typically, you'll do one set of 10 to 12 repetitions to begin your program, adjusting up or down based on your particular level of fitness.

D1 EXTENSION: ARMS

To improve the strength, endurance, and coordination of the muscles in this pattern (posterior arm and shoulder), attach one end of the elastic band to a fixed object above your left shoulder. You can also use your left arm, raised toward the ceiling, to anchor the end of the band. Hold the other end of the band in your right hand and position your right arm in the flexion end of D1 (flexion, adduction, and external rotation: "grab seat belt") (figure 3.10, *a-b*, p. 28).

From this starting position, begin a slow and controlled motion to reach down, out, and behind you, ending at the extension end of D1 (extension, abduction, internal rotation: "fasten seat belt").

Remember, good form is more important than how hard you can pull!

Once you've reached the end of D1 extension, begin a slow and controlled return to your starting position. You may find that this eccentric contraction (or negative work) is more difficult.

That makes one repetition. Typically, you'll do one set of 10 to 12 repetitions to begin your program, adjusting up or down based on your particular level of fitness.

D2 FLEXION: ARMS

To improve the strength, endurance, and coordination of the muscles in this pattern (shoulder and upper back), attach one end of the elastic band to a fixed object to your left at floor level. Hold the free end in your right hand and place your arm at your left hip as if you're sheathing a sword (extension, adduction, internal rotation). Take up the slack on the band by wrapping it around your hand or by stepping or turning a little farther away from it (figure 3.11, *a-b*, p. 29).

From this starting position, begin a slow and controlled motion to reach up and away from your body, as if wielding the sword above your head, ending at the flexion end of D2 (flexion, abduction, external rotation).

Once you've reached the end of D2 flexion, begin a slow and controlled return to your starting position. You may find this eccentric contraction (or negative work) more difficult.

That makes one repetition. Typically, you'll do one set of 10 to 12 repetitions to begin your program, adjusting up or down based on your level of fitness.

D2 EXTENSION: ARMS

To improve the strength, endurance, and coordination of the muscles in this pattern (chest and shoulder), attach one end of the elastic band to a fixed object above your right shoulder. Hold the free end of the band in your right hand and position your right arm in the flexion end of D2 (flexion, abduction, and external rotation: "drawing the sword") (figure 3.12, *a-b*, p. 29).

From this starting position, begin a slow and controlled motion to reach down and across to your left hip, turning your arm as you go, ending at the extension end of D2 (extension, adduction, internal rotation: "sheathing the sword"). Remember, good form is more important than how hard you can pull!

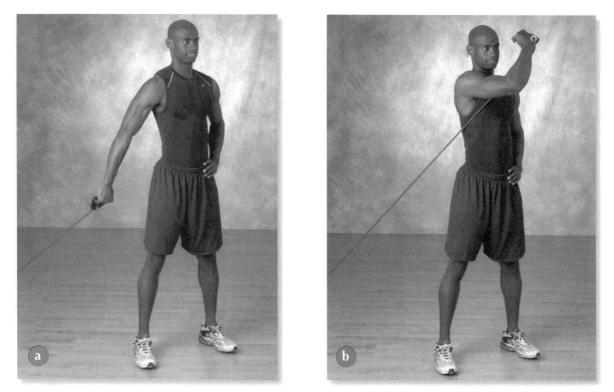

Figure 3.9   Elastic band exercise, D1 flexion, arm. *(a)* Starting position ("fasten seat belt") and *(b)* ending position ("grab seat belt").

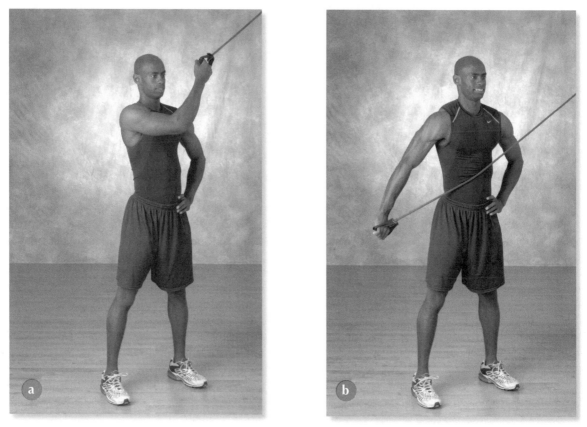

Figure 3.10   Elastic band exercise, D1 extension, arm. *(a)* Starting position ("grab seat belt") and *(b)* ending position ("fasten seat belt").

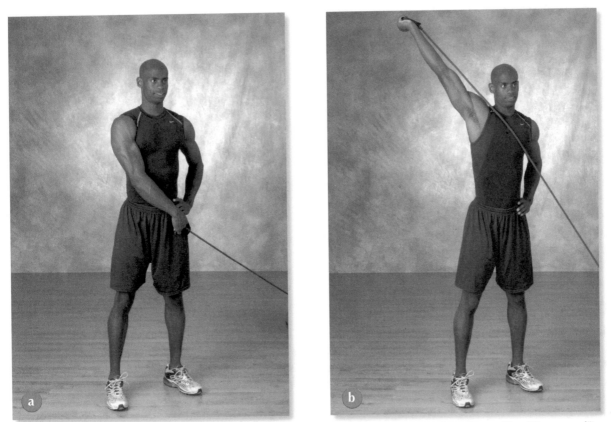

Figure 3.11 Elastic band exercise, D2 flexion, arm. *(a)* Starting position ("sheath sword") and *(b)* ending position ("draw sword").

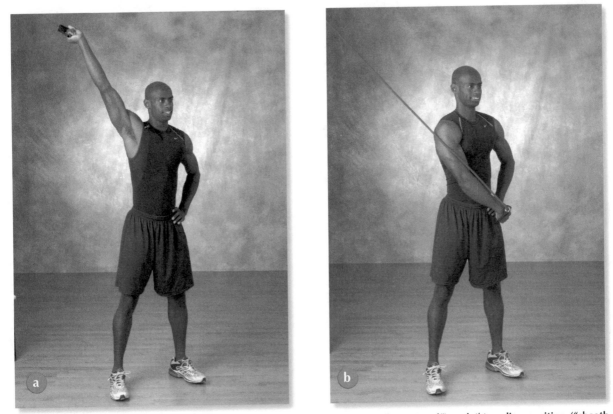

Figure 3.12 Elastic band exercise, D2 extension, arm. *(a)* Starting position ("draw sword") and *(b)* ending position ("sheath sword").

Once you've reached the end of D2 extension, begin a slow and controlled return to your starting position. You may find this eccentric contraction (or negative work) more difficult.

That makes one repetition. Typically, you'll do one set of 10 to 12 repetitions to begin your program, adjusting up or down based on your particular level of fitness.

Strengthening the Legs

Once you have become sufficiently familiar with the spiral patterns for the legs by practicing them as general warm-ups, you can begin to focus on using them for a strength workout. Don't work too hard at the beginning of your program, because you may be too sore the next day. It's best to start slowly and work your way up to a more strenuous routine.

D1 FLEXION: LEGS

To improve the strength, endurance, and coordination of the muscles in this pattern (hip flexors and adductors), attach one end of the elastic band to a fixed object behind you at floor level. Attach the other end to your right ankle in such a way that you will be able to rotate your leg. You can make a large loop in the band, or you can use a loop made for this purpose and found in most gyms.

Stand in such a way that you can shift your weight to your left leg, and hold on to something for stability. Place your leg in extension, abduction, and internal rotation ("toe-off"). Adjust your stance to take up the slack on the band (figure 3.13, a-b).

From this starting position, begin a slow and controlled motion, as if you were performing a soccer kick, ending at the flexion end of D1 (flexion, adduction, external rotation). Your goal is to complete this spiral motion with ease and grace. If you can't, adjust your starting position to reduce the resistance on the band.

Once you've reached the end of D1 flexion, begin a slow and controlled return to your starting position. You may find this eccentric contraction (or negative work) more difficult. Be sure to keep your back from arching by focusing on making the motion happen at your hip joint.

That makes one repetition. Typically, you'll do one set of 10 to 12 repetitions to begin your program, adjusting up or down based on your particular level of fitness.

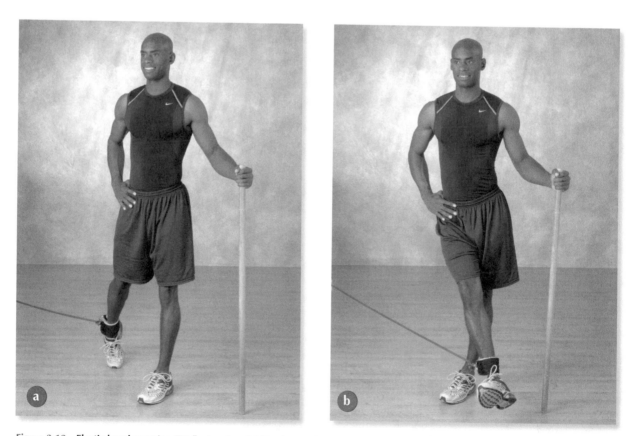

Figure 3.13　Elastic band exercise, D1 flexion, leg. (a) Starting position ("toe-off") and (b) ending position ("soccer kick").

D1 EXTENSION: LEGS

To improve the strength, endurance, and coordination of the muscles in this pattern (hip extensors and abductors), attach one end of the elastic band to a fixed object in front and to your left at floor level. Attach the other end to your right ankle such that you will be able to rotate your leg. You can make a large loop in the band, or use a loop made for this purpose and found in most gyms.

Stand in such a way that you can shift your weight to your left leg, and hold on to something for stability. Place your leg in flexion, adduction, and external rotation ("soccer kick"). Adjust your stance to take up the slack on the band (figure 3.14, a-b).

From this starting position, begin a slow and controlled motion, kicking your leg behind you to the right and ending at D1 extension (extension, abduction, and internal rotation: "toe-off"). Be sure to keep your back from arching by focusing on making the motion happen at your hip joint.

Once you've reached the end of D1 extension, begin a slow and controlled return to your starting position. You may find this eccentric contraction (or negative work) more difficult.

That makes one repetition. Typically, you'll do one set of 10 to 12 repetitions to begin your pro-gram, adjusting up or down based on your level of fitness.

D2 FLEXION: LEGS

To improve the strength, endurance, and coordination of the muscles in this pattern (hip flexors and abductors), attach one end of the elastic band to a fixed object behind and to your left at floor level. Attach the other end to your right ankle in a way that allows you to rotate your leg. You can make a large loop in the band, or use a loop made for this purpose and found in most gyms.

Stand in such a way that you can shift your weight to your left leg, and hold on to something for stability. Place your leg in extension, adduction, and external rotation ("5th position"). Adjust your stance to take up the slack on the band (figure 3.15, a-b, p. 32).

From this starting position, begin a slow and controlled motion, ending up with the right leg in the "snowplow" at the flexion end of D2 (flexion, abduction, internal rotation). Your goal is to complete this spiral motion with ease and grace. Swing the leg from the hip joint and try to keep your pelvis and torso from twisting. If you can't, adjust your starting position to reduce the resistance on the band.

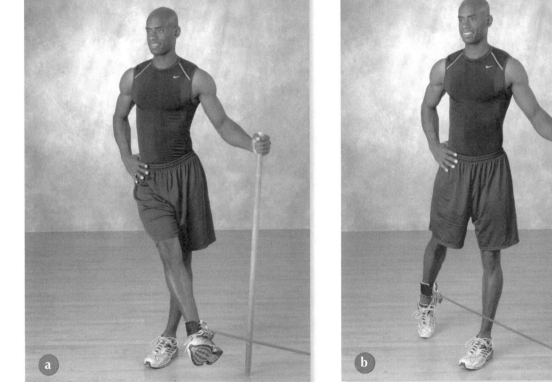

Figure 3.14   Elastic band exercise, D1 extension, leg. *(a)* Starting position ("soccer kick") and *(b)* ending position ("toe-off").

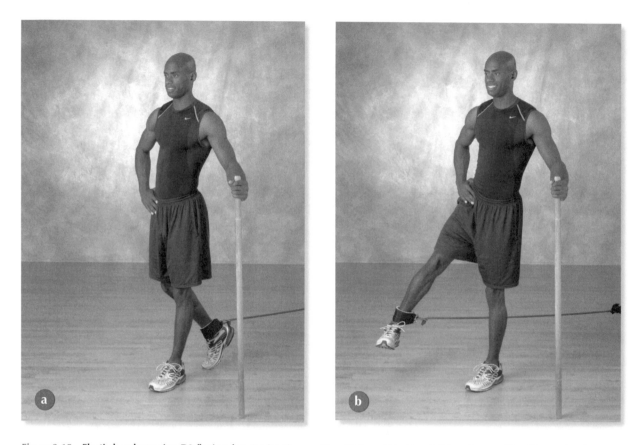

Figure 3.15 Elastic band exercise, D2 flexion, leg. *(a)* Starting position ("5th position") and *(b)* ending position ("snowplow").

Once you've reached the end of D2 flexion, begin a slow and controlled return to your starting position. You may find this eccentric contraction (or negative work) more difficult. Be sure to keep your back from arching by focusing on making the motion happen at your hip joint.

That makes one repetition. Typically, you'll do one set of 10 to 12 repetitions to begin your program, adjusting up or down based on your particular level of fitness.

D2 EXTENSION: LEGS

To improve the strength, endurance, and coordination of the muscles in this pattern (hip extensors and adductors), attach one end of the elastic band to a fixed object in front and to your right at floor level. Attach the other end to your right ankle such that you will be able to rotate your leg. You can make a large loop in the band, or use a loop made for this purpose and found in most gyms.

Stand in such a way that you can shift your weight to your left leg, and hold on to something for stability. Place your leg in flexion, abduction, and internal rotation ("snowplow"). Adjust your stance to take up the slack on the band (figure 3.16, *a-b*).

From this starting position, begin a slow and controlled motion, kicking your leg behind and across your midline, turning your leg out and ending at D2 extension (extension, adduction, external rotation: "5th position").

Once you've reached the end of D2 extension, begin a slow and controlled return to your starting position. You may find this eccentric contraction (or negative work) more difficult.

That makes one repetition. Typically, you'll do one set of 10 to 12 repetitions to begin your program, adjusting up or down based on your particular level of fitness.

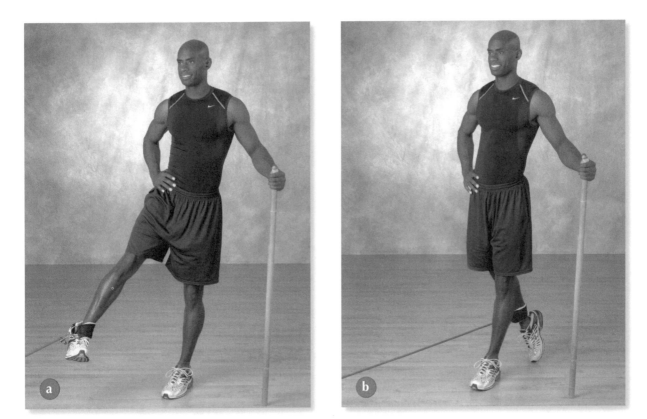

Figure 3.16 **Elastic band exercise, D2 extension, leg.** (a) **Starting position ("snowplow") and** (b) **ending position ("5th position").**

The Stretches

In part I, we looked at the various types of stretching and the importance of using good biomechanics during stretching. We also discussed the background of facilitated stretching and the details for implementing it. Finally, we explored how to use the spiral patterns for stretching and strengthening.

In part II, we show you, step by step, how to stretch each major muscle in the body, both singly and in groups. Chapter 4 covers the hips and legs; chapter 5 is devoted to the shoulder and arm; and chapter 6 details stretches for the neck and torso.

Decision to Use Spiral Patterns or Single-Plane Stretches

PNF techniques were developed as patterns of spiral movement to increase strength, coordination, and flexibility through entire ranges of motion. Facilitated stretching is based on these principles but focuses on increased flexibility and coordination, not necessarily on the development of strength.

When should you use patterns, and when should you use single-muscle, single-plane stretches? We use the spiral–diagonal patterns as a way to increase the flexibility and coordination of groups of muscles that act together. Using these three-dimensional patterns, we stretch groups of muscles simultaneously, thereby gaining greater benefit in a shorter amount of time compared with the single-plane stretches.

We can also use the patterns as an evaluative tool to determine which muscles in a synergistic group are limiting motion, exhibiting weakness, or not firing in the proper sequence. Once these deficiencies are identified, we can modify the patterns to focus on improving the muscular function that needs work.

We use single-plane stretches when we want to develop flexibility or awareness in a specific muscle or muscle group. Single-plane stretches can also be used as an adjunct to soft tissue therapy. For instance, you can use these stretches for relaxing hypertonic (too tight) muscles to reduce the discomfort of deep massage or trigger point work, or in conjunction with deep friction work to release adhesions within or between muscles. (See chapter 7 for more on this.)

Three-Step Stretching Sequence

The three-step stretching sequence was introduced in chapter 2; we place it here also, before presenting the stretches, to remind you of the principal steps in stretching.

1. The stretcher actively lengthens the muscle to be stretched (target muscle).

2. The stretcher isometrically contracts the target muscle for 6 seconds.

3. The stretcher actively stretches the target muscle to a new range of motion.

Organization of Stretches

We've divided each chapter into single-plane stretches and spiral–diagonal patterns, although you may find yourself mixing patterns and single stretches when the need arises. The format for the stretches provides you with the information you need to do them effectively and safely.

Each muscle group is presented as follows:

▪ Anatomy, including the origin, insertion, and action of the muscle(s), with illustrations

▪ Functional assessment for normal range of motion

▪ Detailed stretching instructions, with illustrations

▪ Self-stretching instructions, where appropriate, with illustrations

Safety Reminders

Some exercise descriptions require special safety notes. Those are indicated with special symbols. The symbols you see throughout the exercises in part II are explained here. Please adhere to these special notes and cautions when doing any stretch.

 Stop movement. An isometric contraction is one in which no movement occurs. The stretcher begins slowly and builds the contraction as you, the partner, provide matching resistance, only to your level of strength. Don't allow the stretcher to overpower you. In some cases, the stretcher may be using only 10% of his or her strength, in other cases, 100%. It all depends on how strong you are in relation to the stretcher. Once the stretcher has achieved the proper level of isometric contraction, hold it for 6 seconds.

Don't push or pull. The partner should *rarely push or pull* to deepen the stretch.

Stretch pain free. Facilitated stretches should *always be pain free*. If the stretcher experiences pain, try repositioning the limb or use less force during the isometric contraction of the target muscle. If pain persists, don't use facilitated stretching for that particular muscle until you've determined why it's causing pain.

CHAPTER

Stretches for the Lower Extremity

Flexibility in the hips and legs is important to success in most sports. When a muscle is chronically shortened, it cannot develop its full power when called upon to contract. In addition, a chronically short muscle limits range of motion. Consider the runner's gait. Short, tight hamstrings will cause the quadriceps to work harder to accomplish a full stride because they are pulling against the internal resistance of the hamstrings. This extra work fatigues both muscle groups, setting the stage for lackluster performance and for injury.

The stretches in this chapter will help you develop flexibility in the major muscles of the hips and legs, which will contribute to improved athletic performance and more comfort in your daily activities.

Hip Extensors: Hamstrings and Gluteus Maximus

Anatomy

Chronically shortened hamstrings can contribute to low back pain, knee pain, and leg length differences. They can also restrict stride length in walking or running, can cause the quads to overwork, and are more susceptible to injury. Runners often have short, weak hamstrings.

The gluteus maximus is a powerful hip extensor. It can be involved in low back pain, especially if it's hypertonic (too tight), or if it's weak or dysfunctional as a result of injury, overuse, or lack of exercise. For example, the normal muscle activation sequence for hip extension is initiated by gluteus maximus, with the assistance of biceps femoris, and followed by contraction of the low-back muscles (to help stabilize the lumbar spine). If the normal contraction sequence is altered, the erector spinae will contract first, followed by gluteus maximus and hamstrings. This pattern places excessive stress on the lumbar spine, which may lead to back pain.

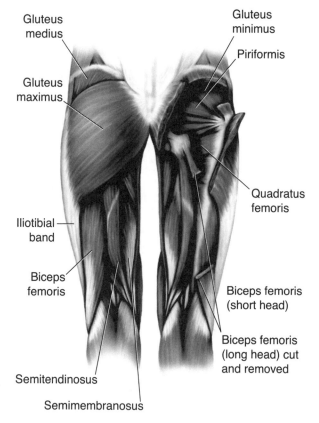

Muscle	Origin	Insertion	Action
Gluteus maximus	Medial one-third of the posterior ilium, just inferior to the posterior iliac crest, lateral sacrum, coccyx, and the sacrotuberous ligament	The posterior aspect of the iliotibial band and the gluteal tuberosity of the femur	Powerfully extends the hip, especially from a flexed position Lower fibers assist lateral rotation of the femur
HAMSTRINGS			
Biceps femoris	Long head: ischial tuberosity Short head: linea aspera of femur	Head of the fibula	Long head: hip extension Both heads: knee flexion, lateral rotation of lower leg with knee flexed
Semimembranosus, semitendinosus	Ischial tuberosity	Semimembranosus: posteromedial tibial condyle Semitendinosus: anterior proximal tibial shaft (pres anserine)	Hip extension Knee flexion Medial rotation of lower leg with knee flexed

Functional Assessment

Check range of motion (figure 4.1). Hip flexion to 90 degrees with the leg straight is optimal. If range is less than 90 degrees, do facilitated stretching for the hamstrings.

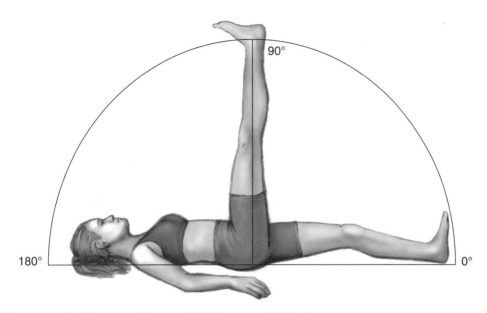

90°

180°

0°

Figure 4.1 **Hip flexion to 90 degrees with the knee straight is ideal.**

Hamstrings Stretch, Straight Leg, Supine, With a Partner

This is an effective, general stretch for the hamstrings that increases hip flexion. The most common compensation during the hamstrings stretch is for the stretcher to lift the hip off the table. This is usually an unconscious attempt to recruit the more powerful gluteus maximus to make up for weak hamstrings. By making sure that both hips stay flat on the table, we ensure that the hamstrings are isolated.

1. The stretcher is supine. She lifts her right leg, with her knee straight, as high as possible. As the partner, your job is to remind the stretcher to keep her knee straight as she lifts. This lengthens the right hamstrings to their pain-free end of range.

2. Position yourself to offer resistance to the isometric contraction of the hamstrings (figure 4.2). The stretcher must keep her hips flat on the table during the entire sequence. You may need to work with the stretcher on body awareness until she is able to stabilize her hips properly before performing this stretch. The stretcher may bend her left knee and rest her foot flat on the table instead of having her left

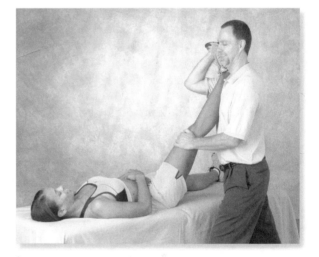

Figure 4.2 **Starting position of the straight leg hamstrings stretch (right leg). The stretcher actively deepens the stretch with no assistance from the partner.**

leg outstretched, if this is a more comfortable position.

3. Direct the stretcher to begin slowly to attempt to push her heel toward the table, isometrically contracting the hamstrings for 6 seconds. ("Push against me as if you're trying to put your heel on the table.")

HIP EXTENSORS

4. After the isometric push, the stretcher relaxes and inhales deeply. During this time, maintain the leg in the starting position.

 5. As she exhales, the stretcher contracts the hip flexors (quads and psoas) to lift the leg higher, keeping her knee straight. This deepens the hamstrings stretch. As the stretcher lifts her leg higher, remind her to keep her knee straight.

6. Now move into the new position to once again offer resistance.

7. Repeat two to three times.

Hamstrings Stretch, Bent Knee, Supine, With a Partner

This is a better stretch for people with very short hamstrings. Once they've achieved more flexibility, you can use the straight leg stretch. The bent-knee position focuses the isometric effort on the distal hamstrings and can be used as an adjunct to soft-tissue work in this area.

1. The stretcher lies supine and lifts her thigh to flex her hip to 90 degrees, with the knee bent.

2. Stabilize the thigh in this vertical position while the stretcher straightens the lower leg as far as possible, without pain. This lengthens the hamstrings to their pain-free end of range (figure 4.3a).

3. Position yourself to offer resistance to the isometric contraction of the hamstrings, at the same time making sure that the stretcher keeps her hips on the table. The stretcher must keep her hips flat on the table during the entire sequence. You may need to work with the stretcher on body awareness until she is able to stabilize her hips properly before performing this stretch.

4. Direct the stretcher to begin slowly to attempt to push her heel toward the table, as if bending the knee, isometrically contracting the hamstrings for 6 seconds. ("Keep your thigh where it is, and try to bend your knee by pushing your heel toward the table.")

5. After the isometric push, the stretcher relaxes and inhales deeply. During this time, maintain the leg in the starting position.

 6. As she exhales, the stretcher contracts her quadriceps to straighten the leg farther. This deepens the hamstrings stretch. As the stretcher

straightens her leg, gently hold the thigh in the 90-degree position (figure 4.3b).

7. Repeat two to three times.

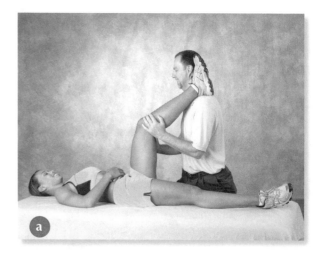

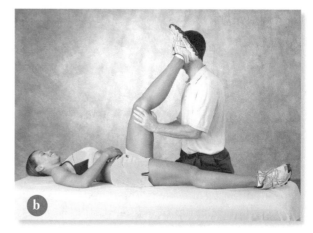

Figure 4.3 *(a)* **Starting position, bent knee hamstrings stretch (right leg).** *(b)* **The stretcher actively deepens the stretch with no assistance from the partner.**

Hamstrings Self-Stretch, Supine, With Stretching Strap

For self-stretching, the sequence of steps is the same as for assisted stretching, but the partner is replaced by a towel, a stretching strap, or an upright object such as a doorjamb.

1. Lie on your back and lift your left leg as high as possible, keeping your knee straight. Keep both hips flat on the floor during the entire sequence. You may bend your right knee and rest your foot flat on the floor, instead of having your right leg

outstretched, if this is a more comfortable position. Use a towel or stretching strap wrapped around the arch of your foot, close to the heel to provide resistance to the hamstrings contraction. The strap simply replaces the partner (figure 4.4).

2. Begin slowly to attempt to push your left heel toward the floor, isometrically contracting the hamstrings for 6 seconds. After the isometric push, relax and inhale deeply. During this time, maintain the leg in the starting position.

3. As you exhale, contract your hip flexors (quads and psoas) to lift the leg higher, keeping your left knee straight. This deepens the hamstrings stretch. Do not pull on the strap to deepen the stretch.

4. Repeat two to three times.

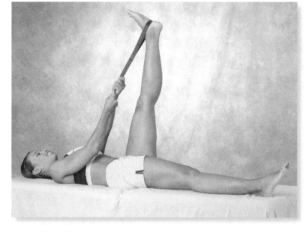

Figure 4.4   Hamstrings self-stretch with a stretching strap.

Hamstrings Self-Stretch, Standing

1. Stand with your right leg and foot stretched out comfortably in front of you, with just your heel on the floor (your toes are up). Bend forward from your hips (no stooping) until you feel a stretch developing in your right hamstrings (figure 4.5a).

2. From this starting position, the floor provides resistance as you try to drag your right heel back toward you, isometrically contracting your hamstrings for 6 seconds. After the isometric push, relax and inhale deeply. During this time, maintain the leg in the starting position.

3. As you exhale, lean forward until you once again feel a stretch in your right hamstrings (figure 4.5b).

4. Repeat two to three times.

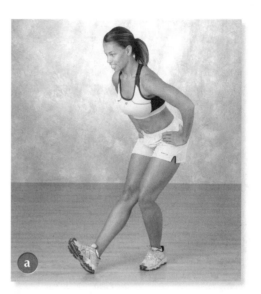

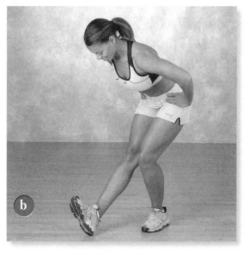

Figure 4.5   (a) Starting position of the hamstrings standing self-stretch. (b) Deepening the stretch.

Gluteus Maximus Stretch, Supine, With a Partner

The gluteus maximus is a strong mover of the hip and is often overworked as part of a cocontraction pattern with the iliopsoas. This stretch is useful for normalizing the tone of gluteus maximus.

1. The stretcher is supine. She lifts her left leg, with the knee bent, as close to her chest as possible.

HIP EXTENSORS

HIP EXTENSORS

Both hips stay flat on the table to ensure that she is stretching the muscle and not just rotating her pelvis. As the partner, assist to passively move her thigh closer to her chest until she feels a stretch in the gluteus maximus or until you reach the end of her comfortable range of motion. Some stretchers will experience a painful pinch in the front of their hip when the leg is brought toward the chest. You can usually eliminate this by wrapping your hands around the thigh near the bent knee and tractioning the thigh toward the ceiling before flexing it toward the chest.

2. Position yourself to offer resistance to the isometric contraction of the gluteus maximus. To avoid stressing the knee joint, place your left hand behind the joint, between the thigh and the leg (figure 4.6, *a & b;* see detail photo).

3. Direct the stretcher to begin slowly to push against your hand to attempt to bring her leg toward the table. ("Push against me as if you're trying to put your thigh back down on the table.") She holds this isometric contraction of the gluteus maximus for 6 seconds.

4. After the isometric push, the stretcher relaxes and inhales deeply. During this time, maintain the leg in the starting position.

5. As she exhales, passively bring the stretcher's thigh closer to her chest to deepen the stretch of the gluteus maximus.

6. Repeat two to three times.

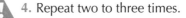

Gluteus Maximus Self-Stretch, Supine

1. Lie on your back and bring your left knee to your chest as far as is comfortable, keeping both hips flat on the table. You may need to place your hands behind your knee and pull your thigh toward you before you feel the stretch on the gluteus maximus (figure 4.7).

2. From this starting position, push against your clasped hands as if you're going to put your thigh back down on the table (or floor). Hold this isometric contraction of the gluteus maximus for 6 seconds. After the isometric push, relax and inhale deeply. During this time, maintain the leg in the starting position.

3. As you exhale, pull your thigh closer to your chest, deepening the stretch on the gluteus maximus.

4. Repeat two to three times.

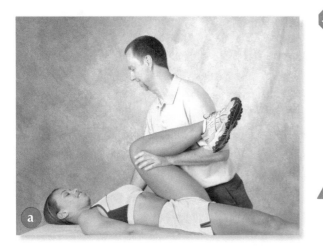

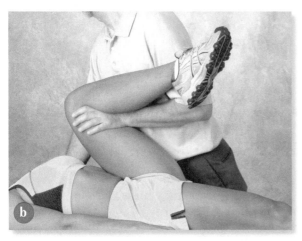

Figure 4.6 *(a)* **Starting position of gluteus maximus stretch.** *(b)* **Hand placement.**

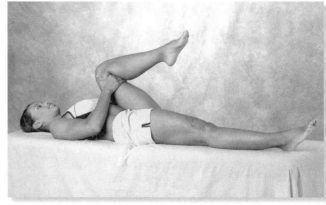

Figure 4.7 **Starting position for the gluteus maximus self-stretch.**

Hip Rotators: Piriformis

Anatomy

The piriformis is one of six deep lateral hip rotators, all of which insert on some portion of the greater trochanter. When these muscles are hypertonic, they contribute to a toe-out gait, commonly seen in dancers, and they restrict internal rotation of the hip. Stretching the piriformis also stretches the other lateral rotators. Although the piriformis is considered to be a lateral rotator of the hip, it may be more important as a postural muscle, acting to stabilize the spine, due to its attachment on the sacrum, and to maintain pelvic balance in conjunction with the psoas (Myers 1998).

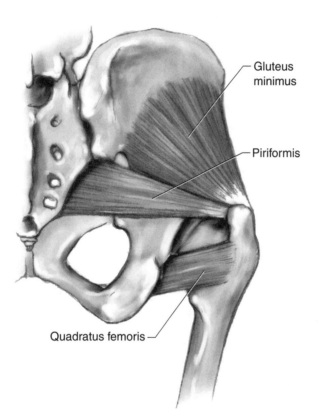

Gluteus minimus

Piriformis

Quadratus femoris

Muscle	Origin	Insertion	Action
Piriformis	Anterior sacrum	Superior aspect of greater trochanter	Lateral rotation of femur
			Assists abduction of femur, especially when hip is flexed
			May act as medial rotator when hip is hyperflexed
			Helps stabilize hip joint

HIP ROTATORS

HIP ROTATORS

Functional Assessment

Because of its importance as a postural muscle, one should always consider the piriformis when investigating causes of low back pain. With the client standing relaxed, in bare feet, check for level iliac crests, anterior superior iliac spines (ASIS), and posterior superior iliac spines (PSIS). Also note whether one PSIS is anterior compared with the other. Imbalance in these areas is common with piriformis syndrome.

With the client supine, compare lateral rotation of the legs. Excessive lateral rotation (45 degrees or more) indicates piriformis shortening on that side.

Tightness in the lateral rotators, including the piriformis, is a common cause of sciatic pain. The sciatic nerve exits the sciatic notch of the ilium and travels through these muscles on its way to the posterior thigh (figure 4.8). When the muscles are hypertonic, they can squeeze the nerve, causing irritation and pain. You may be able to differentiate this type of sciatic pain , called piriformis syndrome, from true sciatica by determining where the pain begins. If shooting or burning pain originates at the lumbar spine and travels through the buttock and down the leg, the cause is likely to be true sciatica. If this type of pain begins in the buttocks and travels down the leg, it's likely to be piriformis syndrome, which responds well to massage and stretching. A leg length difference can also contribute to piriformis syndrome.

Morton's foot or overpronation can result in excessive medial rotation and adduction of the thigh during running and walking, causing the piriformis to be overworked as it attempts to counteract medial rotation. This may lead to the muscle's being "locked long" in a chronic eccentric contraction.

Piriformis Stretch, Supine, With a Partner

This stretch is used to improve medial rotation of the femur. You may have to experiment a little with the starting position of this stretch because each stretcher will feel the muscle stretch in a different position.

1. The stretcher is supine, with his left hip and knee flexed to 90 degrees and drawn up toward the right shoulder; the right leg rests on the table. Be sure the stretcher keeps his sacrum on the table to anchor the origin of the piriformis. The stretcher then rotates his left thigh laterally by bringing his left foot closer to his right shoulder while maintaining flexion at the hip.

2. Place one hand on the stretcher's lateral knee and the other at his lateral ankle to assist him in finding the leg position that begins to stretch the piriformis. Be sure the stretcher keeps his sacrum on the table. From this starting position, offer resistance to the isometric contraction (figure 4.9).

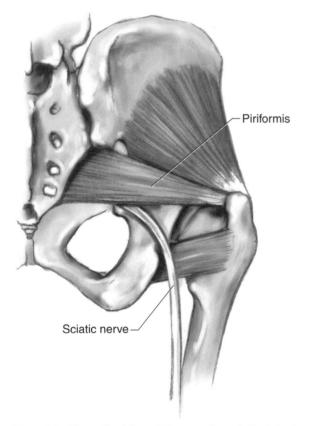

Figure 4.8 **The path of the sciatic nerve through the lateral rotators.**

Piriformis

Sciatic nerve

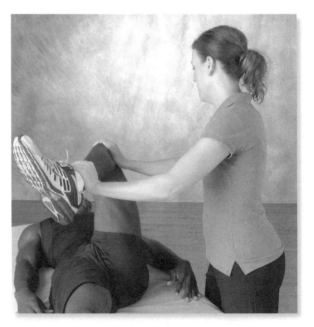

Figure 4.9 **Starting position of the piriformis stretch.**

3. Direct the stretcher to begin slowly to attempt to push his leg toward you diagonally (with equal pressure at both the knee and ankle), isometrically contracting the piriformis for 6 seconds.

4. After the isometric push, the stretcher relaxes and inhales deeply. As he relaxes, maintain the leg in the starting position.

5. As he exhales, he contracts his hip flexors and adductors to deepen the piriformis stretch. You may assist by gently pushing to assist hip flexion and adduction, then by adding more lateral rotation to deepen the stretch.

6. Repeat two to three times.

Piriformis Stretch, Prone, With a Partner

This is an alternate position to increase piriformis length. Some stretchers report feeling more of a stretch in this position, others prefer the supine stretch.

1. The stretcher is prone on the table. He bends his right knee to approximately 90 degrees and externally rotates his thigh (rolls his leg toward the floor), being sure to keep both hips flat on the table. This lengthens the piriformis to its end range.

2. Stand at the stretcher's right side and place your left hand on his foot or medial ankle; your right hand rests lightly on his sacrum (figure 4.10).

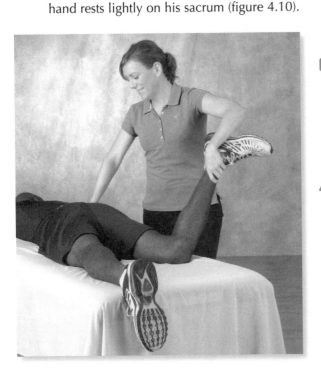

Figure 4.10 **Starting position of the prone piriformis stretch.**

Direct the stretcher to begin slowly to push against your left hand, attempting to bring his leg across his midline. He holds this isometric contraction of the piriformis for 6 seconds. Make sure there is no pain at the medial knee during the isometric phase. If the stretcher experiences medial knee pain, adjust your hold by bringing your right hand to support the medial knee. If this does not eliminate the pain, use a different stretch for the piriformis.

3. After the isometric push, the stretcher relaxes and inhales deeply. As he relaxes, maintain the leg in the starting position.

4. As he exhales, the stretcher once again rolls the leg toward the floor, deepening the stretch on the piriformis.

5. Repeat two to three times.

Piriformis Self-Stretch, Supine

1. Lie on your back; let your left leg rest on the table while you bend your right knee to about 90 degrees and bring the knee up toward your left shoulder. You want to feel a slight stretch deep in the right buttocks, so you may need to play with the position of the leg until you find the "sweet spot." Try adding a little rotation of the thigh by pulling your ankle closer to you (figure 4.11a, p. 46). Keep your hipbones on the table. Many people experience pain when they try to do this because they are overstretching. Stretch only in the "feels-good" range, and not into discomfort.

2. From this starting position, hold your right leg at the knee and ankle and push your leg away from you diagonally, feeling the muscles work deep in the buttocks. This is an isometric contraction, so don't let your leg actually move from your starting position. Breathe normally and hold the push for 6 seconds, then relax.

3. Stretch by bringing your right knee and leg closer to your left shoulder, using your leg muscles as much as possible to do this and pulling with your arms only at the end. Add a little more rotation by pulling your ankle closer to you. Remember to stay in the comfort zone.

4. As an alternative starting position, you may also cross the right ankle over the left knee, then bring the left knee toward the left shoulder, being sure to keep the hipbones in contact with the floor or table to begin the stretch of the right piriformis. Hold your left leg behind the knee with both hands (figure 4.11b).

HIP ROTATORS

HIP ROTATORS

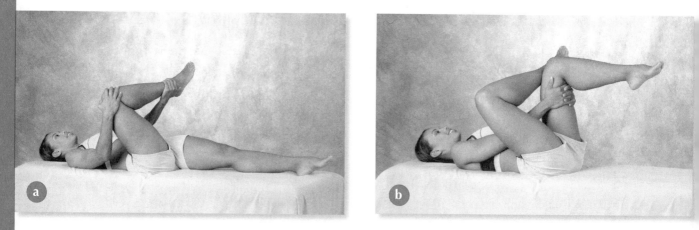

Figure 4.11 **Piriformis self-stretch.** *(a)* **Starting position.** *(b)* **Alternate starting position.**

5. Then push your right leg away from you, using your left knee to resist the motion. Remember, this is an isometric contraction, so don't actually move your right leg. Hold the push for 6 seconds, then relax.

6. Stretch by bringing your right knee and leg closer to you, using your leg muscles as much as possible to do this, and pulling with your left leg and arms only at the end. Remember to stay in the comfort zone.

Piriformis Self-Stretch, Sitting

1. Sit at the edge of a chair and cross your left ankle over your right knee. Keeping your spine lengthened, bend at the hips (no stooping) until you feel a stretch deep in the buttocks. Many people experience pain when they try to do this because they are overstretching. Stretch only in the "feels-good" range, and not into discomfort (figure 4.12).

2. From this starting position, push your left ankle into your right thigh, isometrically contracting the piriformis, for 6 seconds. It may also feel good to push against the inside of your left knee with your left hand. After the isometric push, relax and inhale deeply.

3. As you exhale, sit up tall and bend forward from the hips to deepen the piriformis stretch. Repeat two to three times.

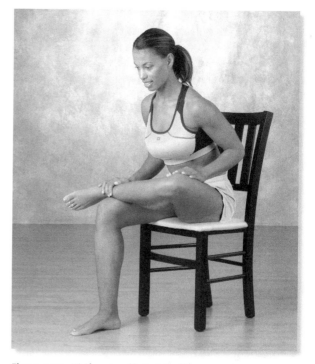

Figure 4.12 **Piriformis self-stretch, sitting.**

Hip Abductors

Anatomy

The primary abductors of the hip are the tensor fasciae latae (TFL) and the gluteus medius and minimus. These muscles not only abduct the hip; they also stabilize it during weight-bearing activities. Tightness in these muscles can contribute to pelvic imbalances, which can cause pain not only in the hips, but also in the low back and the knee.

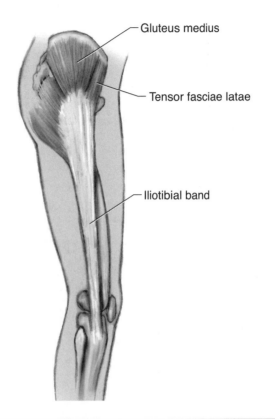

Gluteus medius

Tensor fasciae latae

Iliotibial band

Muscle	Origin	Insertion	Action
HIP ABDUCTORS			
Tensor fasciae latae (TFL) and iliotibial (IT) band	Iliac crest, just posterior to anterior superior iliac spine	Iliotibial band, which then inserts at lateral tibial condyle (Gerdy's tubercle)	Prevents knee from collapsing during movement Assists abduction, medial rotation, and flexion of hip Assists knee extension
Gluteus medius	Just below crest of ilium, between the anterior and posterior gluteal lines Its posterior one-third is covered by gluteus maximus	Posterior superior aspect of greater trochanter	Primary abductor of hip Anterior fibers assist medial rotation and flexion of hip Stabilizes pelvis during walking or running When left leg is in swing phase (non-weight bearing), right gluteus medius contraction prevents pelvis from tilting down on left
Gluteus minimus	Deep to gluteus medius, attaching along lateral surface of the ilium, between the anterior superior iliac spine and the greater sciatic notch	Anterior superior greater trochanter	Abduction of hip Anterior fibers assist medial rotation and flexion of hip Assists gluteus medius in stabilizing the pelvis

HIP ABDUCTORS

Functional Assessment

The leg is normally able to swing across the midline of the body about 30 degrees if slight adjustments are made in the position of the legs. This motion can be limited by excessive tightness in the hip abductors. Because these muscles also function as knee stabilizers, via the iliotibial (IT) band, knee problems can develop when they are hypertonic (too tight).

To test for this, have the stretcher lie on his side, with the knee of the top leg tucked behind the knee of the other leg (figure 4.13). Excessive tightness in the hip abductors prevents this position and can lead to problems such as IT band syndrome.

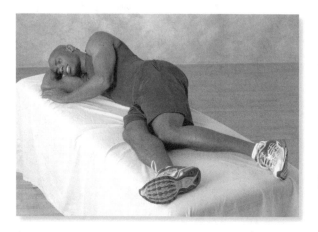

Figure 4.13 Abductor tightness test (modified Ober's test). Excessive tightness in the hip abductors prevents this position.

Iliotibial band syndrome is an overuse injury that occurs when a tight IT band rubs over the lateral femoral condyle. It's often found in cyclists and novice runners who overpronate. The pain is normally experienced just proximal to the lateral knee but may also be found at the IT band insertion on the tibia. Figure 4.14 shows the areas of pain. Tightness in the band can be caused by a tight TFL or gluteus medius, which pulls on the band, or by a hypertrophied vastus lateralis, which bulges under the band and stretches it.

Gluteus medius and minimus are frequently hypertonic and develop trigger points; these may cause pain that mimics sciatica or sacroiliac joint dysfunction.

Hip Abductors Stretch, Supine, With a Partner

This stretch is used to improve adduction at the hip.

1. The stretcher is supine, his right leg flat on the table; his left leg is placed over the right, knee bent, and foot flat on the table. (This keeps the left leg from interfering with right leg adduction.) He adducts the right leg across the midline as far as possible, keeping the kneecap pointed toward the ceiling to prevent the leg from rolling. This lengthens the right abductors to their end range.

2. Place one hand on the lateral knee of the right leg and stabilize the opposite hip with the other hand to provide resistance to the isometric contraction of the abductors (figure 4.15).

3. Direct the stretcher to begin slowly to try to push his leg against your hand, isometrically contracting the abductors for 6 seconds.

4. After the isometric push, the stretcher relaxes and inhales deeply. As he relaxes, maintain the leg in the starting position.

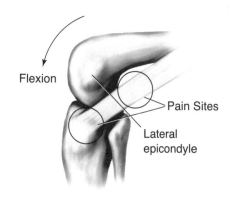

Figure 4.14 Typical pain sites for iliotibial band syndrome.

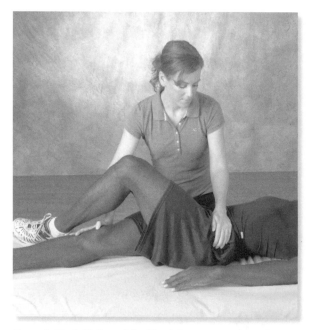

Figure 4.15 Initiation of the hip abductors stretch, supine.

5. As he exhales, the stretcher pulls his leg farther across the midline, deepening the abductor stretch.

6. Repeat two to three times.

Hip Abductors Stretch, Side-Lying, With a Partner

This stretch is used to improve adduction at the hip.

1. The stretcher is side-lying at the edge of the table, top leg hyperextended and hanging over the edge of the table; the bottom leg is bent and the knee as close to the chest as possible, for comfort and stability in the low back. The hips are stacked vertically on top of each other. The stretcher contracts his adductors to pull the top leg toward the floor, lengthening the abductors to their end range. If the stretcher experiences any low back pain in this position, he may bend forward from the waist to round his low back while keeping his leg hanging off the edge of the table.

2. Stand behind the stretcher to offer support, and stabilize his hip with one hand. Place your other hand across the lateral aspect of the knee joint to offer resistance to the isometric contraction of the abductors (figure 4.16).

3. Direct the stretcher to begin slowly to try to push his leg toward the ceiling, isometrically contracting the abductors for 6 seconds.

4. After the isometric push, the stretcher relaxes and inhales deeply. As he relaxes, allow the leg to drop toward the floor.

5. As he exhales, the stretcher pulls his leg toward the floor, deepening the abductor stretch even farther.

6. Repeat two to three times.

Hip Abductors Self-Stretch, Sitting

This is a modification of a stretch position often used in group exercise classes.

1. Sit comfortably on the floor or a stretching mat with your left leg straight out in front of you. Cross your right leg over your left, with the right knee bent and the right foot against the outside of your left knee. Sit up tall and twist your torso to the right as far as is comfortable, place your left elbow or upper arm (or both) against the outside of your right knee, and steady yourself with your right hand behind you (figure 4.17).

2. From this starting position, push your right knee against your left arm, isometrically contracting the hip abductors for 6 seconds. As an added benefit, this will also engage your oblique abdominal muscles.

3. After the isometric push, relax and inhale, and as you exhale, use your leg muscles (adductors) to pull your right leg more toward the left, deepening the stretch on your abductors. Add a gentle push with your left arm as long as it feels good to do so.

4. Repeat two to three times.

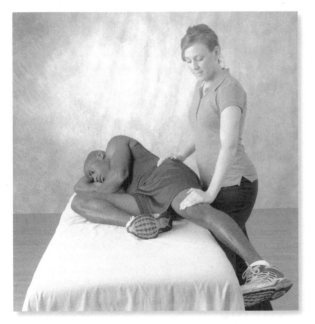

Figure 4.16　Initiation of the side-lying hip abductors stretch.

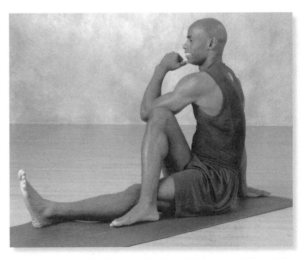

Figure 4.17　Initiation of the hip abductors self-stretch, sitting.

HIP ABDUCTORS

Hip Abductors Self-Stretch, Standing

1. Stand sideways to and about arm length from a wall or other vertical object (post, doorjamb, etc.). Place your right hand against the wall, and cross your right leg behind your left as far as you can with your right foot on the floor. Lean your right hip toward the junction of the floor and the wall as far as you can go comfortably to feel a stretch along your right hip (figure 4.18).

2. From this starting position, attempt to drag your right leg toward the wall, using the floor to provide resistance to this isometric contraction of your hip abductors. After 6 seconds, relax and inhale deeply. As you exhale, lean your right hip closer toward the floor, stretching the right abductors.

3. Repeat two to three times.

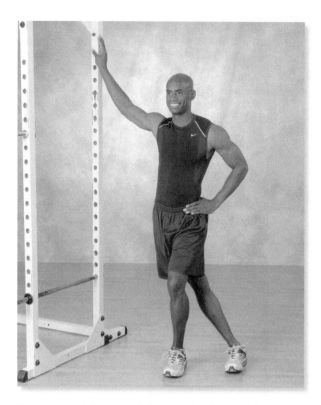

Figure 4.18 Initiation of the standing hip abductors self-stretch.

HIP ABDUCTORS

Hip Adductors

Anatomy

When you bring your legs together (toward your midline), you are using your adductor muscles. The adductor muscles can be divided into the short adductors (pectineus, adductor brevis, and adductor longus) and the long adductors (adductor magnus and gracilis). We've provided one illustration showing all the adductors.

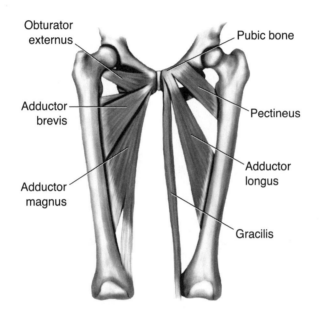

Muscle	Origin	Insertion	Action
SHORT ADDUCTORS			
Pectineus	Superior pubic ramus	Between the lesser trochanter and linea aspera of posterior femur	Hip flexion Assists adduction and lateral rotation of hip
Adductor brevis and longus	Anterior pubis	Linea aspera of posterior femur	Adduction of hip Assists flexion and lateral rotation of hip
LONG ADDUCTORS			
Adductor magnus	Pubic ramus, ischial tuberosity	Vertically along linea aspera of posterior femur and to the adductor tubercle of the medial femur	Powerful adduction of hip The anterior fibers (Origin on pubic ramus) assist hip flexion The posterior fibers (Origin on ischial tuberosity) assist hip extension
Gracilis	Anterior pubis	Medial proximal tibia (pes anserine)	Adduction of hip Assists knee flexion and medial rotation of tibia when knee is flexed

Functional Assessment

Check the range of motion. Normally, the legs should be able to abduct 45 to 50 degrees from the midline (figure 4.19). If this range is limited, the reason is often tight adductors. Use facilitated stretching to increase this range.

The adductors also variously assist hip flexion, hip extension, and lateral rotation, and they help to stabilize the legs in running. They are commonly much tighter in men than in women. Groin pulls are often related to fatigue or improper stretching of the adductor longus.

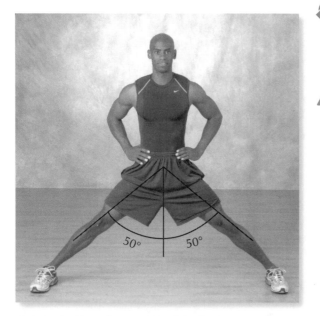

Figure 4.19 Normal range of hip abduction is 45 to 50 degrees from the midline. Limited range is usually due to tight adductors.

Hip Adductors Stretch, Supine, With a Partner

This stretch is used to increase abduction. Occasionally stretchers experience abductor cramping during this stretch. If this occurs, stop and stretch the abductors, then come back to the adductor stretch.

1. The stretcher is supine. Keeping both hips flat on the table, and without arching his back, he abducts his right hip as far as he can, keeping the knee straight and the kneecap pointed toward the ceiling (this prevents rotation of the leg). He may hook his left heel over the edge of the table to keep his left leg from sliding across the table. In this position, the adductors on the right are at the end of their range.

2. Standing at the right side of the table, between the table and the stretcher's leg, support the lower leg with your left hand and place your right hand across the medial aspect of the knee. This position prevents stress to the medial collateral ligament during the isometric phase (figure 4.20). Ask the stretcher to begin slowly to attempt to bring his right leg toward the midline, isometrically contracting the adductors for 6 seconds.

3. After the isometric push, the stretcher relaxes and inhales deeply. During this time, maintain the leg in the starting position.

4. As he exhales, ask him to abduct his hip farther, deepening the stretch of the adductors. Be sure he keeps his leg from rolling laterally by asking him to keep his kneecap pointing toward the ceiling.

5. Repeat two to three times. After the final stretch, help the stretcher bring his leg back to the table. This helps prevent possible groin strain.

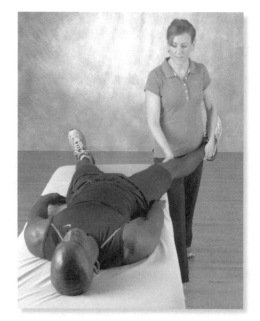

Figure 4.20 Initiation of the supine hip adductors stretch.

Hip Adductors Self-Stretch, Standing

This stretch is an adaptation of a common adductors stretch.

1. To stretch the right adductors, assume a side-lunge position, being careful not to bend the left knee beyond 90 degrees, keeping the right leg straight, foot flat on the floor. All your weight is on your left leg (figure 4.21).

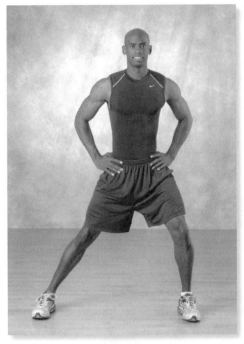

Figure 4.21   **Standing adductors self-stretch.**

2. From this starting position, attempt to pull your right leg toward your midline, using the floor to provide resistance to this movement. After the 6-second isometric contraction, deepen the stretch by sinking lower into your left leg.

Hip Adductors Self-Stretch, Supine, With Stretching Strap

1. Lie on your back on the floor or a stretching mat with both legs out straight and together. Loop one end of a stretching strap around your right foot. Keeping both hips and your back flat on the floor, use your leg muscles (abductors) to move your right leg away from your midline as far as is comfortable, keeping your kneecap pointed toward the ceiling to avoid rotating your leg and keeping your back flat on the floor. Take up the slack on the stretching strap (figure 4.22).

2. From this starting position, try to drag your leg back to the middle, isometrically contracting your adductors against the stretching strap for 6 seconds, breathing normally. Keep your back and left leg as relaxed as possible.

3. After the isometric effort, relax and breathe, and as you exhale, use your abductors to move your leg farther from your midline, deepening the stretch on your adductors. Remember to keep hips and back flat on the floor.

4. Repeat two to three times.

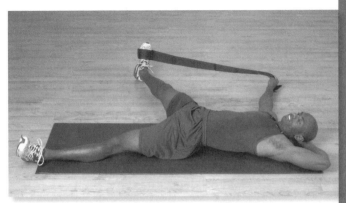

Figure 4.22   **Supine adductors self-stretch with a stretching strap.**

Hip Adductors Self-Stretch, Sitting

This position focuses more on the short adductors.

1. Sit with your back straight, knees bent, and the soles of your feet together. Pull your legs as close to the floor as you can using your leg muscles. This lengthens your short adductors.

2. Place your arms or hands against the inside of your knees, then attempt to bring your knees together against your own resistance, isometrically contracting your short adductors (figure 4.23). Hold the contraction for about 6 seconds, breathing normally.

3. After the isometric effort, relax and breathe, and as you exhale, use your leg muscles to pull your legs closer to the floor, stretching your adductors.

4. Repeat two to three times.

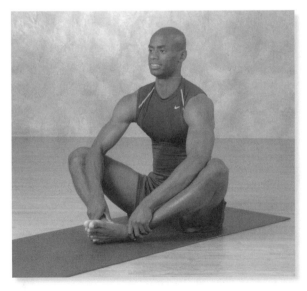

Figure 4.23   **Sitting adductors self-stretch.**

HIP ADDUCTORS

Hip Flexors: Quadriceps Group

Anatomy

The quadriceps consist of four muscles and are powerful extensors of the knee. One of the quads, the rectus femoris, also crosses the hip joint and acts as a hip flexor, assisting the psoas. Chronically short quads can contribute to low back pain. The quadriceps are usually involved in any type of knee pain or instability.

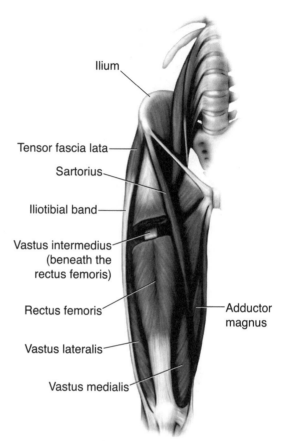

Ilium

Tensor fascia lata

Sartorius

Iliotibial band

Vastus intermedius
(beneath the
rectus femoris)

Rectus femoris

Vastus lateralis

Vastus medialis

Adductor
magnus

Muscle	Origin	Insertion	Action
QUADRICEPS			
Rectus femoris	Anterior inferior iliac spine and upper margin of acetabulum	Patella and via the patellar ligament to tibial tuberosity	Knee extension Assists hip flexion
Vastus medialis, lateralis, and intermedius	Medialis and lateralis: linea aspera of posterior femur Intermedius: anterior and lateral shaft of femur	Patella and via the patellar ligament to tibial tuberosity	Knee extension

Functional Assessment

Check range of motion. The quadriceps extend (straighten) the knee.

▮ *Knee extension*—The stretcher is seated, with legs dangling over the edge of the table. As the stretcher straightens the lower leg, the arc of motion should be smooth and the knee should extend to 0 degrees or beyond into a few degrees of hyperextension (figure 4.24, *a* & *b*).

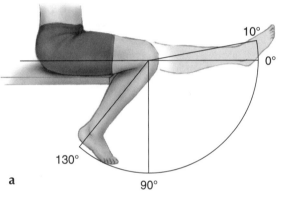

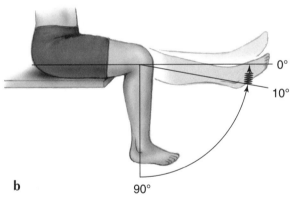

Figure 4.24   Normal range of knee extension. *(a)* The quadriceps should fully extend the knee. *(b)* The arc of motion should be smooth, with no hesitation or jerkiness.

▮ *Knee flexion*—While on her stomach, the stretcher should be able to bring the heel to the buttock, with a little help from you (figure 4.25). If range is limited, the reason may be tight quads, which will be somewhat uncomfortable as you press the heel toward the buttock. Limitation may also be due to the bulk of the hamstrings and calf muscles. Facilitated stretching works quite well here if the limitation is due to tight quads.

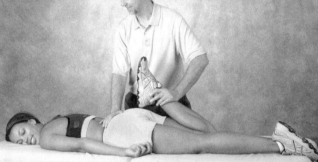

Figure 4.25   **The stretcher should be able to bring her heel to her buttock with a little help.**

⊙ Quadriceps Stretch, Prone, With a Partner

This stretch is used to improve knee flexion.

⚠ 1. The stretcher lies prone, with the knee flexed as far as possible. Because of the bulk of the hamstrings and calf muscles, the stretcher will be unable to stretch the quads to her end of range. Gently push against the leg to bring the heel closer to the buttocks, but only until the stretcher feels the quads beginning to stretch (stretch barrier). Keep the lower leg aligned with the thigh so as not to stress the knee joint. This is the pain-free end of range. If this position

HIP FLEXORS

causes any low back discomfort, stop and place a pillow under the stretcher's hips to reduce the stress on the low back and begin again. Or, you may want to have the stretcher contract her abdominal muscles to stabilize and flatten her low back (a pelvic tilt). This position can also eliminate low back discomfort.

2. Position yourself to offer resistance to the isometric contraction of the quads by placing your hands or shoulder against the stretcher's shin (figure 4.26). The stretcher must keep her hips flat on the table (or on the pillow) during the entire sequence. You may need to work with the

stretcher on body awareness until she is able to stabilize her hips properly before performing this stretch.

3. Direct the stretcher to begin slowly to try to straighten her leg, isometrically contracting the quads for 6 seconds.

4. After the isometric push, the stretcher relaxes and inhales deeply. During this time, maintain the leg in the starting position.

5. As she exhales, the stretcher rests and allows you to offer assistance by pushing on the leg, deepening the quad stretch. Occasionally, the hamstrings will go into spasm at this point, usually because the stretcher is unconsciously contracting them to assist the stretch. You may want to gently rest one hand on the hamstrings to be sure they are not activating.

6. Repeat two to three times.

Quadriceps Self-Stretch, Standing

This is a modification of a commonly used quadriceps stretch.

1. Stand comfortably and use a stationary object to help you stabilize as you bend your left knee and lift your heel toward your buttocks. Hold your left leg or foot with your left hand, keeping your low back flat and being careful to bring your heel toward the center of your buttock and not toward the outside of your hip, as this may stress your knee ligaments (figure 4.27a).

2. From this starting position, attempt to straighten your left leg against your own resistance, isometrically contracting your quadriceps for 6 seconds. After the isometric push, relax and inhale, and as you exhale, pull your heel closer to your buttock.

3. As your flexibility improves, you may find that your heel can easily reach your buttock. If this is the case, then your goal with each stretch is to bring your thigh to a more vertical position so that the knee points directly to the floor, all the while keeping your low back flattened to prevent hyperextension of the lumbar spine (figure 4.27b).

4. Repeat two to three times.

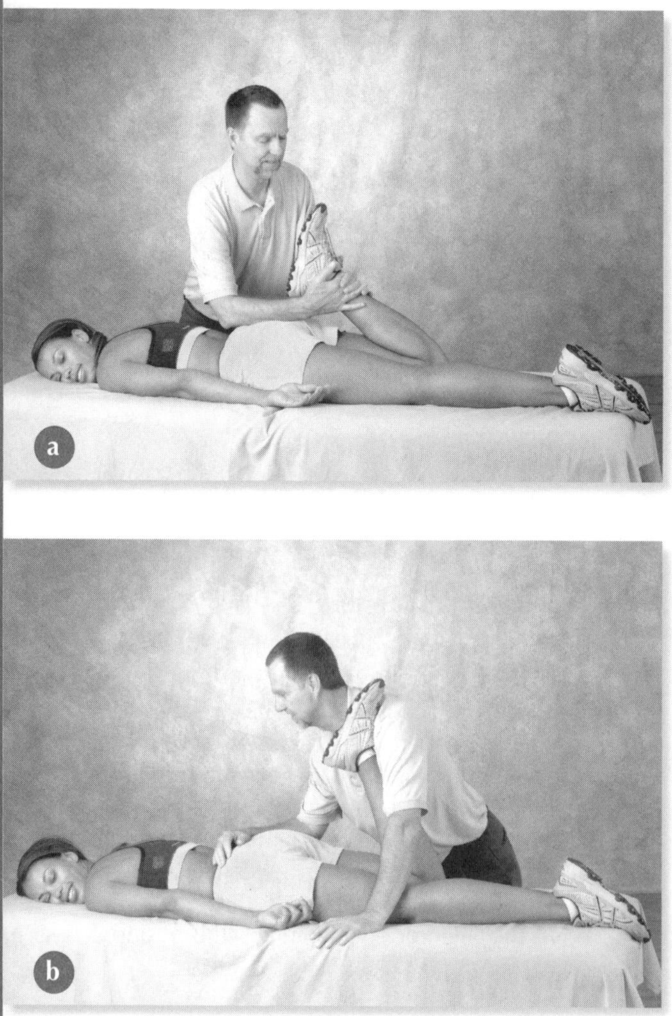

Figure 4.26 Initiation of the quadriceps stretch. (a) Use your hands, fingers interlaced, or (b) use your shoulder.

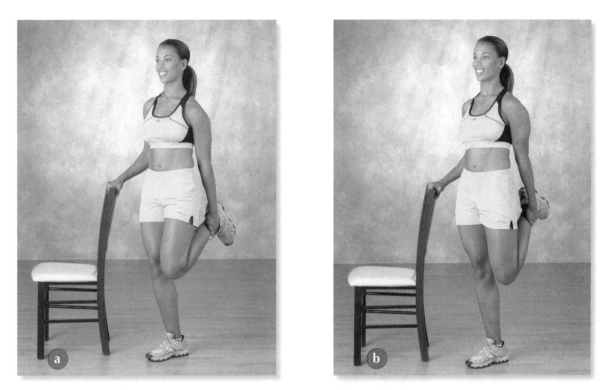

Figure 4.27   Quadriceps standing self-stretch. *(a)* Heel toward buttock. *(b)* If your heel can easily reach your buttock, then try to point your knee directly toward the floor.

HIP FLEXORS

Hip Flexors: Psoas and Iliacus

Anatomy

The iliopsoas is the primary hip flexor. Because of its attachment along the lumbar spine, it affects the angle of the lumbar curve. A psoas that is too tight can cause an increase in the curve, which leads to swayback and low back pain. However, sometimes a tight psoas will flatten the lumbar curve, which can also lead to low back pain. For a more detailed discussion of this seeming contradiction, see Tom Myers' article, "Poise: Psoas-Piriformis Balance" (1998).

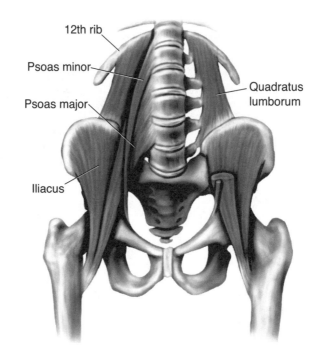

Muscle	Origin	Insertion	Action
Iliopsoas	Psoas: anterior lumbar vertebrae	Lesser trochanter of femur	Flexion and lateral rotation of the femur
	Iliacus: inner surface of ilium		Experts disagree on whether it acts as an abductor or adductor

HIP FLEXORS

Functional Assessment

Check hip range of motion as well as tightness in the psoas and quadriceps.

▪ *Hip range of motion*—Normal range of flexion (120 degrees) allows the stretcher to bring her flexed knee to her chest. Normal range in extension is approximately 30 degrees (figure 4.28, *a* & *b*).

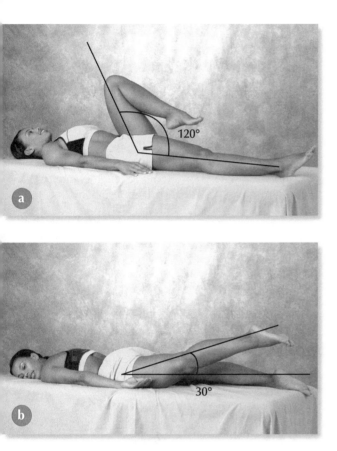

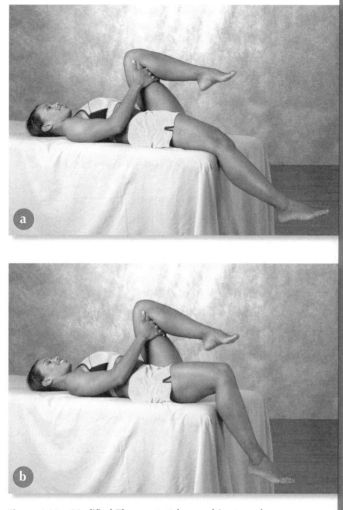

Figure 4.29 Modified Thomas test for quadriceps and psoas tightness. *(a)* The stretcher flexes her left hip and knee, bringing the knee to her chest. The right lower leg extends, indicating a tight quadriceps, and possibly a tight tensor fasciae latae, on the right. *(b)* The right thigh lifts off the table, indicating a tight psoas on the right.

Figure 4.28 Normal range of *(a)* hip flexion and *(b)* hip extension.

▪ *Modified Thomas test*—To check for tightness in the psoas or quadriceps (or both), the stretcher lies supine with the lower legs dangling off the edge of the table, then lifts the left leg, knee to chest. Check to see whether the stretcher's right lower leg straightens. This indicates tight quadriceps (especially rectus femoris) and TFL on the right leg (figure 4.29*a*). If the stretcher's right thigh lifts off the table (figure 4.29*b*), this indicates a tight iliopsoas on the right.

Repeat for the other leg. It's common for both the quads and the iliopsoas to be hypertonic on the same leg. If the quads are too tight, do facilitated stretching for the quads. If the iliopsoas is too tight, do facilitated stretching for the iliopsoas.

Psoas Stretch, Prone, With a Partner

This stretch is used to improve hip extension. The stretcher must keep her hips flat on the table (or on the pillow) throughout this stretch. There will be

HIP FLEXORS

a strong tendency for her to lift her hip as she lifts her leg. You may need to work with the stretcher on body awareness until she is able to stabilize her hips properly before performing this stretch.

1. The stretcher lies prone. If she has any low back discomfort in this position, place a pillow under her hips to take some of the stress off the low back. Or you may want the stretcher to contract her abdominal muscles to stabilize and flatten her low back. This position can also eliminate low back discomfort.

2. The stretcher uses her hip extensors (gluteals and hamstrings) to lift her leg off the table as high as possible, with the knee bent. This lengthens the iliopsoas to its end of range. Remember that normal range of hip extension is only 30 degrees. If the stretcher seems more flexible than that, look for hypermobility in the low back area.

3. Support the leg just above the knee to provide resistance to the isometric contraction of the iliopsoas. Use your hand to support the stretcher (figure 4.30).

4. Direct the stretcher to begin slowly to try to pull her thigh toward the table, isometrically contracting the iliopsoas for 6 seconds. She is not trying to straighten her lower leg. As the stretcher contracts her psoas, she should relax her gluteal muscles, but it's often the case that the gluteal muscles are cocontracting with the psoas. This is an inefficient pattern, to be discouraged. You can help the stretcher eliminate this pattern by having her briefly drop the weight of her leg into your hand prior to the isometric contraction of the psoas. After a few times, the stretcher should be able to do this automatically.

5. After the isometric push, the stretcher relaxes and inhales deeply. During this time, maintain the leg in the starting position.

6. As she exhales, the stretcher contracts the hip extensors to lift her thigh higher, deepening the psoas stretch. Be sure the stretcher keeps her hips flat on the table.

7. Repeat two to three times.

Psoas Self-Stretch, Standing or Kneeling

A widely used standing stretch can easily be modified to become a facilitated stretch for the iliopsoas.

1. Stand with your right leg forward and left leg back, keeping your torso upright and your low back flat.

2. Keeping your left foot flat on the floor, lunge forward with your left hip to lengthen the left iliopsoas. Allow your right knee to bend as you push forward. You should feel the stretch high on the front of the left thigh (figure 4.31).

3. Isometrically contract the left iliopsoas by attempting to pull your left leg forward but keeping the foot anchored on the floor. To avoid an unnecessary cocontraction pattern, be sure your gluteal muscles are relaxed. Maintain the isometric contraction for 6 seconds, then relax.

4. You can now stretch the iliopsoas by pushing the left hip forward again, being sure to maintain an upright posture with your low back flat.

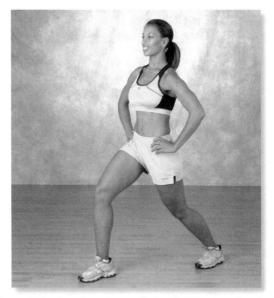

Figure 4.31 Standing psoas self-stretch. Keep your low back flat and focus on feeling the stretch high on the front of your left thigh.

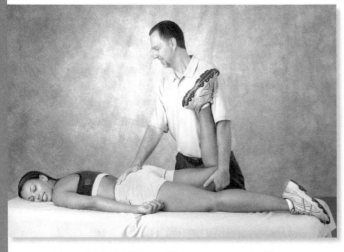

Figure 4.30 Initiation of the prone psoas stretch.

Plantarflexors: Gastrocnemius and Soleus

Anatomy

The gastrocnemius-soleus muscles are also called the triceps surae. They insert into the heel via the Achilles tendon, the strongest tendon in the body. The gastrocnemius is a two-headed muscle that gives the calf its shape. The soleus muscle, which lies underneath the gastrocnemius, is more often the reason for calf tightness.

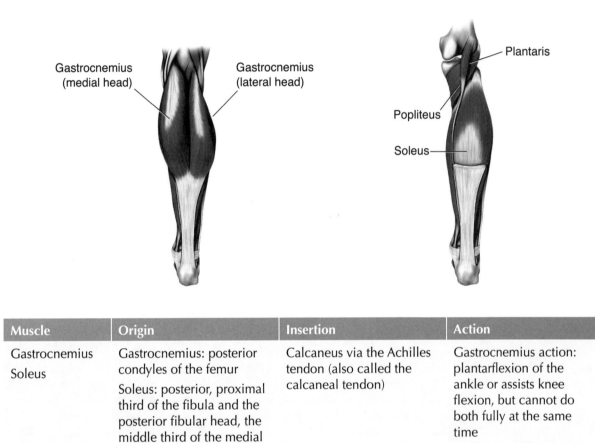

Muscle	Origin	Insertion	Action
Gastrocnemius Soleus	Gastrocnemius: posterior condyles of the femur Soleus: posterior, proximal third of the fibula and the posterior fibular head, the middle third of the medial border of the tibia, and the tendinous arch across the proximal tibia and fibula	Calcaneus via the Achilles tendon (also called the calcaneal tendon)	Gastrocnemius action: plantarflexion of the ankle or assists knee flexion, but cannot do both fully at the same time Soleus action: plantarflexion of the ankle

PLANTARFLEXORS

Functional Assessment

Check range of motion. Dorsiflexion should be approximately 20 degrees (figure 4.32a).

If dorsiflexion is limited, have the stretcher lie prone and flex the knee to 90 degrees and test again (figure 4.32b). Knee flexion relaxes the gastrocnemius and eliminates it as a limiter of dorsiflexion. So if limitation is still present after the knee is flexed, focus the stretching on the soleus. If knee flexion improves dorsiflexion, focus the stretching on the gastrocnemius.

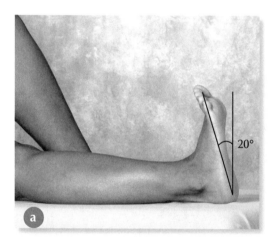

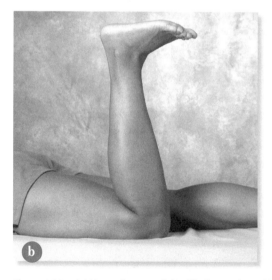

Figure 4.32 *(a)* Normal range of dorsiflexion at the ankle. *(b)* With the knee bent, the gastrocnemius is slack, and any limitation in dorsiflexion is probably due to a tight soleus.

Plantarflexion should be 50 degrees (figure 4.33). Limited plantarflexion may be due to a tight tibialis anterior.

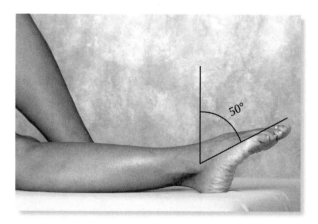

Figure 4.33 **Normal range of ankle plantarflexion is 50 degrees.**

Gastrocnemius Stretch, Prone, With a Partner

1. The stretcher lies prone on the table, with her feet hanging over the edge far enough so that she can fully dorsiflex without interference from the table.
2. The stretcher dorsiflexes one foot (brings the foot toward the knee) as far as possible. This lengthens the gastrocnemius to its end of range.
3. Stand at the end of the table and place the palm of your hand against the stretcher's foot. Use your thigh to support your hand, being sure to maintain good posture (figure 4.34).

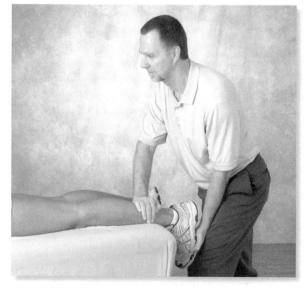

Figure 4.34 **Initiation of gastrocnemius stretch, prone.**

Offer resistance as you direct the stretcher to begin slowly to attempt to plantarflex (push the foot toward you), isometrically contracting the gastrocnemius-soleus for 6 seconds.

4. After the isometric push, the stretcher relaxes and inhales deeply. During this time, maintain the foot in the starting position.

5. As she exhales, the stretcher contracts the tibialis anterior, dorsiflexing the foot and deepening the gastrocnemius stretch.

6. Repeat two to three times.

Gastrocnemius Self-Stretch, Sitting, With Stretching Strap

1. Sit comfortably with your right leg straight, a stretching strap looped around the ball of your foot. If you have enough flexibility, hold the foot in your hands instead of using a stretching strap. Use your leg muscles to bring your foot and toes as close to you as possible (figure 4.35).

2. From this starting position, try to push your foot away from you, isometrically contracting the gastrocnemius for 6 seconds. After the isometric push, relax and inhale, and as you exhale, use your leg muscles again to bring your foot toward you, deepening the stretch on the gastrocnemius.

3. Repeat two to three times.

Soleus Stretch, Prone, With a Partner

This stretch isolates the soleus and is used to improve dorsiflexion.

1. The stretcher lies prone on the table, with one knee flexed to 90 degrees. This position isolates the soleus muscle because it puts the gastrocnemius at a mechanical disadvantage. She then dorsiflexes her foot (brings the foot toward the knee) as far as possible. This lengthens the soleus to its end of range.

2. Support the bent leg with one hand and wrap your other hand around the heel with your forearm resting against the sole of the foot. As another option, sit on the table, interlace your fingers, and place them across the metatarsal arch of the foot (figure 4.36, *a* & *b*).

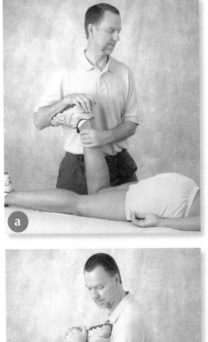

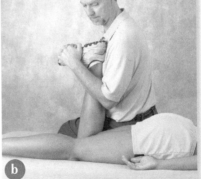

Figure 4.36   Initiation of the soleus stretch. *(a)* Support the bent leg with one hand and wrap your other hand around the heel, with your forearm resting against the sole of the foot. *(b)* Or, sit on the table, interlace your fingers, and place your hands across the metatarsal arch of the foot.

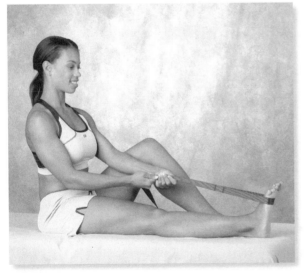

Figure 4.35   Gastrocnemius self-stretch, sitting, with a stretching strap.

PLANTARFLEXORS

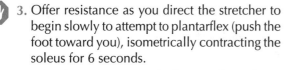

3. Offer resistance as you direct the stretcher to begin slowly to attempt to plantarflex (push the foot toward you), isometrically contracting the soleus for 6 seconds.

4. After the isometric push, the stretcher relaxes and inhales deeply. During this time, maintain the foot in the starting position.

5. As she exhales, the stretcher contracts the tibialis anterior, dorsiflexing the foot and deepening the soleus stretch.

6. Repeat two to three times.

Soleus Self-Stretch, Sitting

1. Sit comfortably with your right knee bent and hold your right foot in your hands. Use your leg muscles to bring your foot and toes as close to you as possible (figure 4.37).

2. From this starting position, try to push your foot away from you, isometrically contracting the soleus for 6 seconds. After the isometric push, relax, inhale, and as you exhale, use your leg muscles again to bring your foot toward you, deepening the stretch on the soleus.

3. Repeat two to three times.

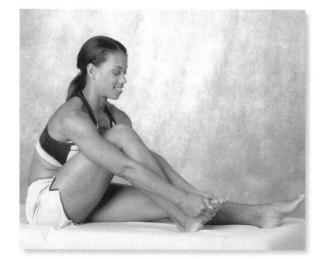

Figure 4.37 **Soleus self-stretch, knee bent.**

PLANTARFLEXORS

Toe Flexors: Flexor Hallucis Longus, Flexor Digitorum Longus

Anatomy

We illustrate and discuss only two of the six toe flexors (flexor hallucis and flexor digitorum longus). The muscle table lists all six toe flexors. With the foot on the ground, flexors hallucis and digitorum longus assist in maintaining balance by keeping the toe pads on the ground. Flexor hallucis longus helps to support the longitudinal arch and exerts a strong propulsion action during the toe-off phase of gait.

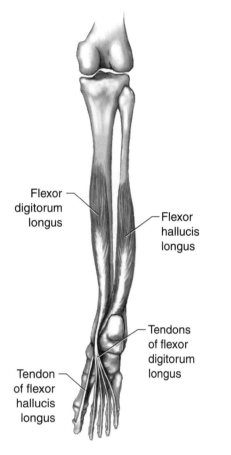

Flexor digitorum longus

Flexor hallucis longus

Tendons of flexor digitorum longus

Tendon of flexor hallucis longus

Muscle	Origin	Insertion	Action
TOE FLEXORS			
Flexor hallucis longus	Inferior two-thirds of the posterior fibula and interosseous membrane	The tendon passes behind the medial malleolus, passes underneath the tendon of flexor digitorum longus, and attaches to the plantar aspect of the distal phalanx of the great toe	Flexes the great toe Assists ankle supination Weak ankle plantarflexion
Flexor hallucis brevis	Medial aspect of the cuboid and the middle and lateral cuneiform bones	The two heads attach to the medial and lateral aspect of the distal phalanx of the great toe Each tendon contains a sesamoid bone	Flexes the great toe

(continued)

Muscle	Origin	Insertion	Action
TOE FLEXORS			
Flexor digitorum longus	Posterior surface of the middle third of the tibia, distal to the popliteal line	The tendon passes behind the medial malleolus, crosses the flexor hallucis longus tendon, then splits into four tendon slips and inserts onto the plantar aspect of the distal phalanges of toes 2-5	Flexes toes 2-5 Assists ankle plantarflexion
Quadratus plantae (also called flexor digitorum accessorius)	Two heads arise from the medial and lateral borders of the inferior aspect of the calcaneus	The muscle spreads out to attach to the tendons of flexor digitorum longus	Assists flexion of toes 2-5
Flexor digitorum brevis	Medial process of the calcaneal tuberosity and the deep surface of the plantar fascia	Splits into four tendons that attach to the plantar aspect of the middle phalanges of toes 2-5	Flexes toes 2-5
Flexor digiti minimi brevis	Base of the fifth metatarsal	Lateral aspect of the base of the proximal phalanx of the fifth toe	Flexes the little toe

Functional Assessment

The normal range of motion of the great toe is approximately 80 degrees of extension and 25 degrees of flexion (figure 4.38). If extension is limited, stretch the flexors.

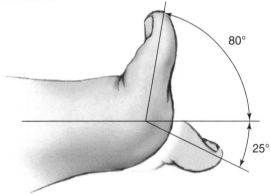

Figure 4.38 Normal range of motion of the great toe: 80 degrees of extension, 25 degrees of flexion.

Toe Flexors Stretch, Prone, With a Partner

This stretch is used to improve extension of the toes.

1. The stretcher lies prone on the table with his right knee flexed to 90 degrees and his toes fully extended (pointing toward the table). This lengthens the toe flexors to their end range.

2. Support the leg with your left hand and cradle the toes lightly with your right (figure 4.39).

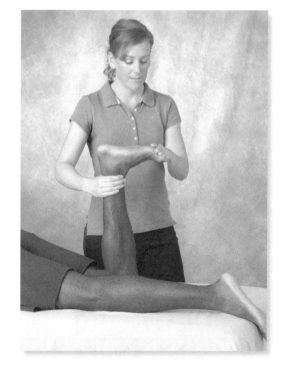

Figure 4.39 **Initiation of the toe flexors stretch.**

3. Offer resistance as you direct the stretcher to try to curl his toes, isometrically contracting the toe flexors for 6 seconds.

4. After the isometric push, the stretcher relaxes and inhales deeply. During this time, maintain the foot and toes in the starting position.

5. As he exhales, the stretcher uses his muscles to pull the toes farther into extension, deepening the stretch on the toe flexors.

6. Repeat two to three times.

Toe Flexors Self-Stretch, Sitting

1. Sit comfortably with your left knee bent. Use your muscles to bend your toes toward you, and hold your toes lightly with your hand (figure 4.40).

2. From this starting position, try to curl your toes, isometrically contracting the flexors for 6 seconds. After the isometric push, relax, inhale, and as you exhale, use your muscles again to bring your toes toward you, deepening the stretch on the flexors.

3. Repeat two to three times.

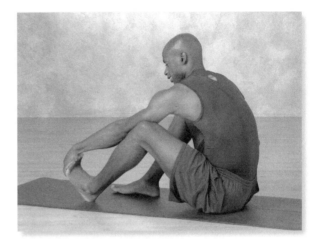

Figure 4.40   **Toe flexors self stretch.**

TOE FLEXORS

DORSIFLEXORS

Dorsiflexors: Tibialis Anterior

Anatomy

When the foot is free to move, tibialis anterior dorsiflexes and inverts it. When the foot is on the ground, tibialis anterior assists in maintaining balance. During walking or running, it helps prevent the foot from slapping onto the ground after heel strike and lifts the foot to clear the ground as the leg is swinging forward.

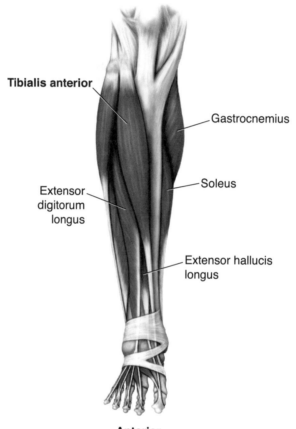

Tibialis anterior

Gastrocnemius

Extensor digitorum longus

Soleus

Extensor hallucis longus

Anterior

Muscle	Origin	Insertion	Action	°
Tibialis anterior	Lateral shaft of tibia, interosseous membrane	Base of fifth metatarsal, first cuneiform	Ankle dorsiflexion Inversion of foot Supports longitudinal arch	

Functional Assessment

Check range of motion (figures 4.32 and 4.33, p. 62). Dorsiflexion of the ankle should be approximately 20 degrees. Plantarflexion of the ankle should be approximately 50 degrees. If range of motion is limited, stretching may be helpful.

Tibialis Anterior Stretch, Supine, With a Partner

This stretch is used to improve plantarflexion.

1. The stretcher lies supine and plantarflexes his right ankle (points toes) using the calf muscles. This lengthens the right tibialis anterior to its end of range.
2. Cup the right heel with your left hand and hold the top of the right foot with your right hand (figure 4.41). When stretching the left side, cup the left heel with your right hand and hold the top of the left foot with your left hand.
3. Direct the stretcher to begin slowly to attempt to pull his foot toward his knee (dorsiflexion), isometrically contracting the tibialis anterior for 6 seconds.
4. After the isometric pull, the stretcher relaxes and inhales deeply. During this time, maintain the foot in the starting position.
5. As he exhales, the stretcher contracts the calf muscles to increase plantarflexion, deepening the tibialis anterior stretch.
6. Repeat two to three times.

Tibialis Anterior Self-Stretch, Sitting

1. Sit comfortably in a chair, with your right ankle crossed over your left knee. Point your foot and toes and hold the top of your foot with your left hand (figure 4.42).
2. From this starting position, try to pull your foot toward your knee, isometrically contracting your tibialis anterior for 6 seconds. After the isometric push, relax, inhale, and as you exhale, use your calf muscles to point your foot and toes again, deepening the stretch on tibialis anterior.
3. Repeat two to three times.

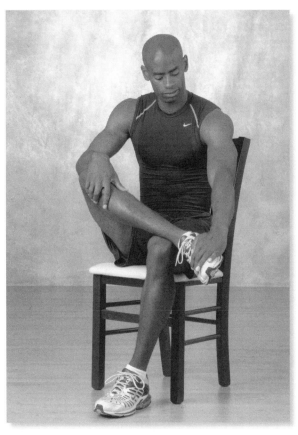

Figure 4.42 Tibialis anterior self-stretch.

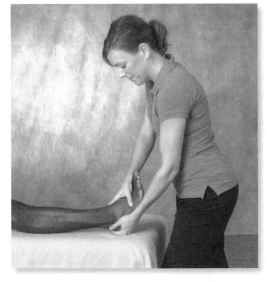

Figure 4.41 Initiation of tibialis anterior stretch, right foot.

DORSIFLEXORS

Toe Extensors: Extensor Hallucis Longus, Extensor Digitorum Longus

Anatomy

We illustrate and discuss only two of the four toe extensors (extensor hallucis longus and extensor digitorum longus). The muscle table lists all four toe extensors. Extensor hallucis longus and extensor digitorum longus help control the speed of descent of the forefoot to the ground following heel strike, preventing the foot from slapping onto the ground. They also contribute to postural stability by controlling posterior sway. With the foot anchored to the ground, they pull the leg forward at the ankle.

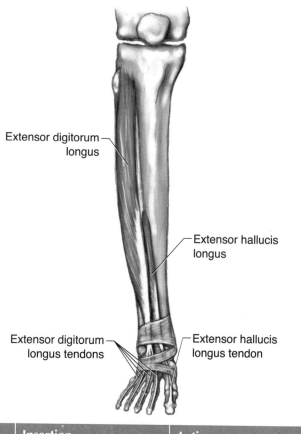

Extensor digitorum longus

Extensor hallucis longus

Extensor digitorum longus tendons

Extensor hallucis longus tendon

Muscle	Origin	Insertion	Action
TOE EXTENSORS			
Extensor hallucis longus	Anteromedial surface of the fibula and the adjacent interosseous membrane	Dorsal aspect of the base of the distal phalanx of the great toe	Extends the great toe Assists ankle dorsiflexion
Extensor hallucis brevis Extensor digitorum brevis	These muscles have a common attachment to the superior aspect of the calcaneus	The medial tendon attaches to the dorsal aspect of the base of the proximal phalanx of the great toe The other three tendons fuse with those of extensor digitorum longus to insert on toes 2-4	Assist in toe extension
Extensor digitorum longus	Lateral condyle of the fibula; proximal two-thirds of the medial fibula; upper part of the interosseous membrane, fascia cruris, and anterior intermuscular septum	Splits into four tendon slips inferior to the extensor retinaculum and inserts onto the dorsal aspect of the middle and distal phalanges of toes 2-5	Extends toes 2-5 Assists ankle dorsiflexion

Functional Assessment

Adequate range of motion in the big toe is essential for normal walking. If extension is limited, then the proper toe-off function will be compromised, and the weight will be shifted to the lateral foot, often with painful results. See figure 4.38 (p. 66) to check flexion and extension range of motion of the great toe. If flexion is limited, stretch the extensors.

Toe Extensors Stretch, Supine, With a Partner

This stretch is used to improve flexion of the toes.

1. The stretcher lies supine with his legs straight or comfortably bolstered under the knees. He curls the toes on his right foot as far as possible. This lengthens the toe extensors to their end range.

2. Stand beside the stretcher's right shin, facing the top of his foot. Support the foot with your left hand and curl your fingers loosely around the stretcher's flexed toes (figure 4.43).

3. Offer resistance as you direct the stretcher to try to straighten his toes, isometrically contracting the extensors for 6 seconds.

4. After the isometric push, the stretcher relaxes and inhales deeply. During this time, maintain the foot and toes in the starting position.

5. As he exhales, the stretcher uses his muscles to pull the toes farther into flexion, deepening the stretch on the extensors.

6. Repeat two to three times.

Toe Extensors Self-Stretch, Sitting

1. Sit comfortably in a chair, with your right ankle crossed over your left knee. Point your foot and curl your toes to stretch the extensors. Use your left hand, wrapped across the toes, to resist as you try to straighten your toes, isometrically contracting the extensors for 6 seconds (figure 4.44).

2. After the isometric push, relax, inhale, and as you exhale, point your foot and curl your toes again, deepening the stretch on the extensors.

3. Repeat two to three times.

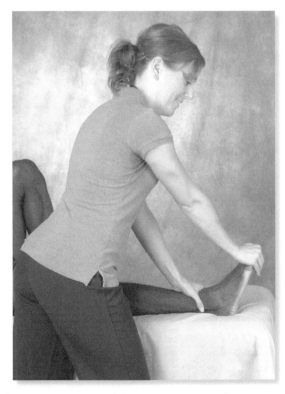

Figure 4.43 Initiation of the toe extensors stretch.

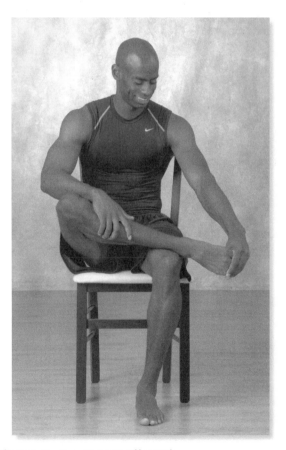

Figure 4.44 Toe extensors self-stretch.

TOE EXTENSORS

Evertors—Peroneal (Fibularis) Group; Invertors—Tibialis Anterior and Posterior

Anatomy

Eversion (pronation) and inversion (supination) of the foot occur with every step in walking or running. Proper function of the evertors and invertors of the foot is critical for maintaining good biomechanics of the foot and ankle, as well as for stabilizing the leg on the foot. Like many of the lower limb muscles, the invertors and evertors often act to control movement rather than initiate it.

The primary evertors of the foot are two of the three peroneal muscles (also known as the fibularis muscles): the peroneus longus and the peroneus brevis. They make up the lateral compartment of the leg. A third evertor, peroneus tertius, when present at all, is found in the anterior compartment with the tibialis anterior.

Although the peroneals are most often considered evertors of the foot, they also function to stabilize the foot, ankle, and leg along with the other muscles of the lower limb.

The primary invertors of the foot are tibialis anterior and posterior. The tibialis posterior is the deepest muscle in the calf. To review the anatomy and actions of the tibialis anterior, see page 68.

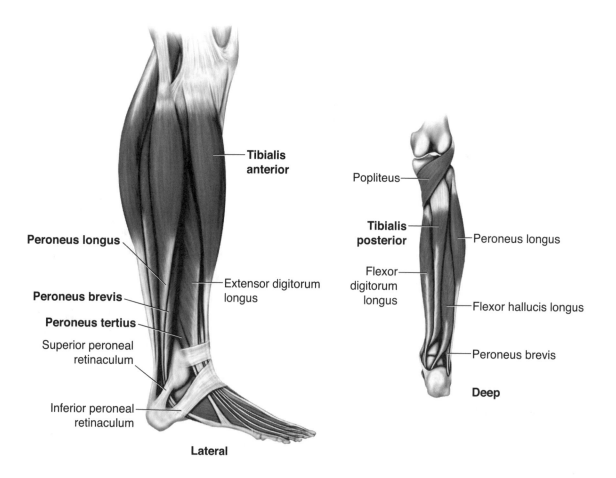

Lateral

Tibialis anterior

Peroneus longus

Peroneus brevis

Peroneus tertius

Superior peroneal retinaculum

Inferior peroneal retinaculum

Extensor digitorum longus

Popliteus

Tibialis posterior

Flexor digitorum longus

Peroneus longus

Flexor hallucis longus

Peroneus brevis

Deep

Muscle	Origin	Insertion	Action
EVERTORS: PERONEAL MUSCLES (ALSO CALLED FIBULARIS)			
Peroneus longus	Proximal two-thirds of lateral fibula	Base of first metatarsal and medial cuneiform	Eversion of foot Assists plantarflexion of foot Stabilizes leg on foot Supports medial arch (in conjunction with tibialis anterior)
Peroneus brevis	Distal two-thirds of lateral fibula (lies deep to peroneus longus)	Peroneal tubercle on lateral aspect of fifth metatarsal	Eversion of foot Assists dorsiflexion
Peroneus tertius (often absent)	Distal half of anterior fibula	Peroneal tubercle on lateral aspect of fifth metatarsal and base of fourth metatarsal	Eversion of foot Assists dorsiflexion
INVERTORS			
Tibialis anterior	Lateral shaft of tibia, interosseous membrane	Base of first metatarsal, first cuneiform	Ankle dorsiflexion Inversion of foot Supports longitudinal arch
Tibialis posterior	Interosseous membrane, medial fibula, and posterolateral tibia	Primarily the navicular and medial cuneiform, and also the cuboid, calcaneus, and bases of the second, third, and fourth metatarsals	Inversion of foot Assists plantarflexion and inversion

Functional Assessment

Check range of motion. Inversion (supination) should be approximately 45 degrees and eversion (pronation) should be approximately 20 degrees (see figure 4.45).

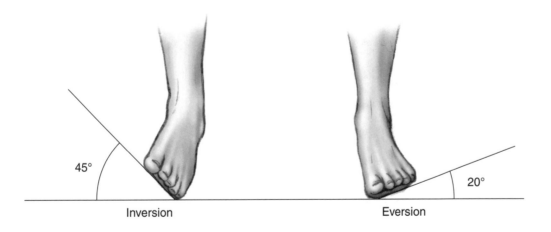

45°

Inversion

20°

Eversion

Figure 4.45   Normal ROM for inversion (supination) is 45° and for eversion (pronation) is 20°.

EVERTORS AND INVERTORS

⊙ Peroneals (Evertors) Stretch, Supine, With a Partner

This stretch is used to increase inversion of the ankle.

1. The stretcher lies supine and inverts his right ankle (turns the sole of his foot toward the midline) by contracting the invertors. The ankle is kept in neutral relative to dorsiflexion or plantarflexion. This lengthens the right peroneals to their end of range.

2. Grasp his lower leg with your right hand to stabilize it, and place your left hand against the lateral side (little-toe side) of the stretcher's right foot (figure 4.46).

3. Direct the stretcher to begin slowly to attempt to turn the sole of his foot out against your hand (eversion), isometrically contracting the peroneals for 6 seconds.

4. After the isometric push, the stretcher relaxes and inhales deeply. During this time, maintain the foot in the starting position.

5. As he exhales, the stretcher contracts the invertors to increase inversion, deepening the peroneal stretch.

6. Repeat two to three times.

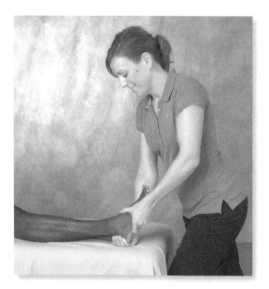

Figure 4.46 **Initiation of the peroneal stretch.**

⊙ Peroneals (Evertors) Self-Stretch, Sitting

1. Sit comfortably in a chair, with your right ankle crossed over your left knee. Bend at the ankle to bring the inside of your foot toward you, as if turning your sole toward your chest (figure 4.47).

2. Grasp the outside of your foot with your left hand and try to turn your foot away from you, isometrically contracting your peroneals for 6 seconds. After the isometric push, relax, inhale, and as you exhale, use your leg muscles to turn your foot toward you again, deepening the stretch on the peroneals.

3. Repeat two to three times.

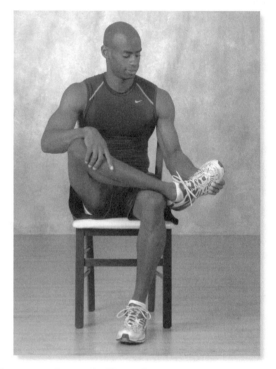

Figure 4.47 **Peroneal self-stretch.**

⊙ Tibialis Posterior (Invertor) Stretch, Supine, With a Partner

This stretch is used to increase eversion of the ankle.

1. The stretcher lies supine and everts his right ankle (turns the sole of his foot away from the midline) by contracting the peroneal muscles (evertors). The ankle is kept in neutral relative to dorsiflexion or plantarflexion. This lengthens the right posterior tibialis to its end of range.

2. Grasp his lower leg with your left hand to stabilize it, and place your right hand against the medial side (big-toe side) of the stretcher's right foot (figure 4.48).

3. Direct the stretcher to begin slowly to attempt to turn the sole of his foot inward against your

hand (inversion), isometrically contracting the posterior tibialis for 6 seconds.

4. After the isometric push, the stretcher relaxes and inhales deeply. During this time, maintain the foot in the starting position.

5. As he exhales, the stretcher contracts the peroneals to increase eversion, deepening the tibialis posterior stretch.

6. Repeat two to three times.

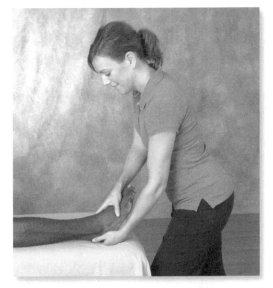

Figure 4.48 **Initiation of tibialis posterior stretch.**

Tibialis Posterior (Invertor) Self-Stretch, Sitting

1. Sit comfortably on the floor or a stretching mat, with your left knee bent and the heel resting on the floor. Use your leg muscles to bend at the ankle and pull your foot out, as if you're turning the sole to the left.

2. From this starting position, wrap your hands around your foot and resist as you try to turn your foot inward, isometrically contracting the invertors for 6 seconds (figure 4.49). After the isometric push, relax, inhale, and as you exhale, use your muscles again to turn the sole of your foot to the left, deepening the stretch on the invertors.

3. Repeat two to three times.

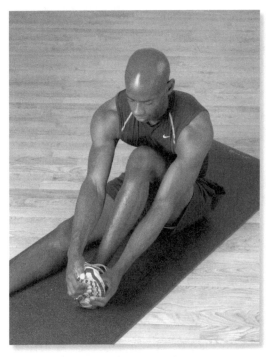

Figure 4.49 **Tibialis posterior self-stretch.**

Spiral–Diagonal Patterns
for the Lower Extremity

Not all the spiral patterns for the leg lend themselves to stretching. For instance, the extension end of the D2 pattern is extremely awkward to carry out. Therefore, we'll be practicing the stretches that are the easiest to learn and use. If you have special circumstances with a particular stretcher, feel free to be creative in developing other stretches based on PNF principles and the patterns for the leg.

Compared to the single-plane stretches, using the patterns requires more concentration from both the stretcher and you. Accordingly, we recommend that you illustrate what you want the stretcher to do by taking him through the pattern passively a few times before attempting to perform the stretch.

Remember, we're trying to improve range of motion at the end of the pattern. We start with the stretcher at the end of his range in all three planes of motion. In the isometric phase, the stretcher is attempting to move toward the opposite three planes, that is, or toward the shortened direction. After the isometric effort, the stretching occurs as the stretcher moves farther in all three planes of motion toward the lengthened direction.

Before proceeding with the exercises, you may find it useful to review, in chapter 3, the leg patterns on pages 23 through 25 as well as the discussion about the change in nomenclature from the previous edition on page 21.

Soccer Kick Stretch (Flexion End of D1)

This stretch is for increasing range of motion in flexion, adduction, and external rotation.

1. The stretcher is supine, with his left leg in as much flexion, adduction, and external rotation as possible. His foot is dorsiflexed and inverted, and the toes are extended. This is the starting position, which lengthens the target muscles to their end range. These include hamstrings (especially biceps femoris), gluteals, TFL, gastrocnemius (especially lateral head), soleus, and peroneals. Demonstrate the pattern passively with the stretcher several times so he knows what you expect him to do during the isometric and the stretching phases.

2. Support and stabilize the leg (figure 4.50). Remember, your hand contacts give the stretcher proprioceptive cues about which way to push or pull. Your hand positions should match your verbal commands.

3. Direct the stretcher to begin slowly to try to initiate the D1 extension pattern, first with internal rotation, then abduction, then extension. ("Begin by rotating, then kick down and out.") The contraction lasts for 6 seconds. Be sure the stretcher keeps both hips flat on the table and initiates the motion from his hip, not from his foot.

4. After the isometric push, the stretcher relaxes and inhales deeply. As he relaxes, maintain the leg in the starting position.

5. As he exhales, the stretcher moves the hip farther into flexion, then into adduction, and then into external rotation. Remember, we want a blend of all three directions to keep moving in a diagonal line. He increases dorsiflexion and inversion of the foot and extension of the toes. Support the leg, but do not push to deepen the stretch.

6. Repeat two to three times.

Soccer Kick Self-Stretch

1. Loop a stretching strap around the sole of your right foot, then wrap the stretching strap around the outside of your ankle and behind your Achilles tendon to the inside of the calf. Lie down on your back, with your legs out straight (figure 4.51, a & b).

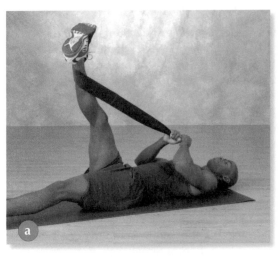

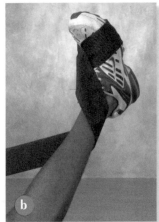

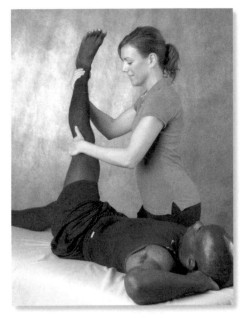

Figure 4.50   **Initiation of the "soccer kick" stretch (D1 pattern). The left leg is flexed, adducted, and externally rotated.**

Figure 4.51   *(a)* **"Soccer kick" self-stretch.** *(b)* **Correct placement of stretching strap around the ankle.**

LOWER EXTREMITY SPIRAL PATTERNS

2. Hold on to the stretching strap, but use your quads to lift your right leg up as high as you can with the knee straight. Then bring the leg across or toward your midline; next, rotate it to the right, so you're looking at the inside of your knee and foot. Take up the slack on the stretching strap. This is the start of the "soccer kick" stretch.

3. Start slowly and try to rotate your leg to the left; then push it down and out, as if you're putting it on the floor to your right. Breathe normally. Use the stretching strap to resist this attempt at motion and hold this isometric contraction for 6 seconds. Then relax and breathe.

4. As you exhale, use your leg muscles, not the stretching strap, to lift your leg higher, across your midline, and to rotate more to the right. This deepens the stretch on the target muscles. Repeat two to three times.

Toe-Off Stretch (Extension End of D1)

This stretch is used to improve range of motion into extension, abduction, and internal rotation. Because the stretcher is prone in this stretch, you may be somewhat confused as to internal versus external rotation. It may help to pay attention only to the thigh and ignore the position of the lower leg and foot when determining which is internal and which is external rotation.

1. The stretcher is prone, with his left knee flexed. Being sure he keeps his hips flat on the table, he lifts his thigh into as much extension, abduction, and internal rotation as possible (the lower leg and foot will be pointing out, away from the midline). Keeping the hips flat on the table helps prevent compensation and muscle substitution. Remember that normal range of hip extension is only 30 degrees. If the stretcher seems more flexible than that, look for hypermobility in the low back area. This starting position lengthens the target muscles to their end range. These include iliopsoas, rectus femoris, the adductors, and the lateral hip rotators. For this stretch, the position of the foot and the toes is not important. The knee is in flexion simply to make it easier for the stretcher to lift his leg off the table. If the stretcher experiences any low back discomfort in this position, stop and place a pillow under his hips to make him more comfortable.

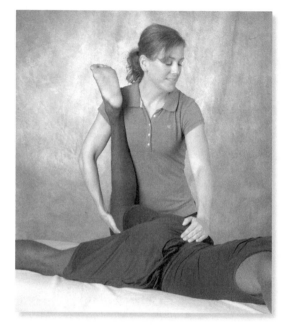

Figure 4.52 Initiation of the "toe-off" stretch (D1 pattern). The knee is bent and the thigh is extended, abducted, and internally rotated. Note that this rolls the leg and foot away from the midline.

2. Support and stabilize the leg, at the same time asking the stretcher to keep both hips on the table (figure 4.52). If the stretcher has enough range of motion, you may be able to support his thigh with your own. If not, use your hand and arm to cradle and support the leg.

3. Direct the stretcher to begin slowly to try to initiate the D1 flexion pattern, with external rotation of the thigh first, then adduction, then flexion. The contraction lasts 6 seconds. ("Begin with rotation, then try to pull down and in.") The stretcher does not try to straighten his knee, only to push his thigh toward the table. The gluteal muscles should be relaxed during the isometric phase.

4. After the isometric push, the stretcher relaxes and inhales deeply. As he relaxes, maintain the leg in the starting position.

5. As he exhales, the stretcher moves his leg farther into extension, then abduction, and then internal rotation. Remember, we want a blend of all three directions to keep moving in a diagonal line. As he lifts, the stretcher must stabilize his pelvis to keep both hips on the table. Support the leg but do not assist to deepen the stretch.

6. Repeat two to three times.

Snowplow Stretch
(Flexion End of D2)

This stretch is used to increase range of motion in flexion, abduction, and internal rotation.

1. The stretcher is supine, with his right leg in as much flexion, abduction, and internal rotation as possible. His foot is dorsiflexed and everted, and the toes are extended. This starting position lengthens the target muscles to their end range. These include gluteals, hamstrings (especially medial), gastrocnemius (especially medial head), soleus, gracilis, adductors, and tibialis posterior. Demonstrate the pattern passively with the stretcher several times so he knows what you expect him to do during the isometric and the stretching phases.

2. Support and stabilize the leg (figure 4.53). Remember, your hand contacts give the stretcher proprioceptive cues about which way to push or pull. Your hand positions should match your verbal commands.

3. Direct the stretcher to begin slowly to try to initiate the D2 extension pattern, with external rotation first, then adduction, then extension. ("Begin with rotation, then kick down and in.") The contraction lasts 6 seconds. Be sure the stretcher keeps both hips flat on the table and initiates the motion from his hip, not from his foot.

4. After the isometric push, the stretcher relaxes and inhales deeply. As he relaxes, maintain the leg in the starting position.

5. As he exhales, the stretcher moves the hip farther into flexion, then into abduction, and then into internal rotation. Remember, we want a blend of all three directions to keep moving in a diagonal line. He increases dorsiflexion and eversion of the foot and extension of the toes. Support the leg but do not push to deepen the stretch.

6. Repeat two to three times.

Snowplow Self-Stretch

1. Loop a stretching strap around the sole of your right foot, then wrap the stretching strap around the inside of your ankle and behind your Achilles tendon to the outside of the calf. Lie down on your back, with your legs out straight (figure 4.54, a & b).

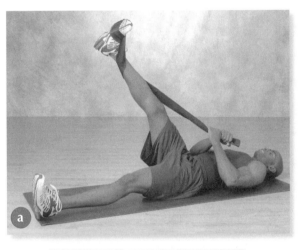
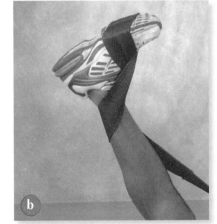

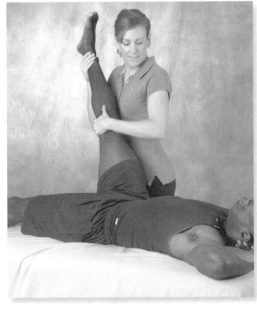

Figure 4.53 Initiation of the "snowplow" stretch (D2 pattern). The right leg is flexed, abducted, and internally rotated.

Figure 4.54 (a) "Snowplow" self-stretch. (b) Correct placement of the stretching strap around the ankle.

2. Hold on to the stretching strap, but use your quads to lift your right leg up as high as you can with the knee straight. Keep both hips flat on the floor. Then bring the leg out away from your midline; then rotate it to the left, so you're looking at the outside of your knee and foot. Take up the slack on the stretching strap. This is the start of the "snowplow" stretch.

3. Start slowly and try to rotate your leg to the right; then push it down and in, as if you're putting it on the floor next to your left leg. Use the stretching strap to resist this attempt at motion and hold this isometric contraction for 6 seconds. Then relax and breathe.

4. As you exhale, use your leg muscles, not the stretching strap, to lift your leg higher, away from your midline, and to rotate more to the left. This deepens the stretch on the target muscles.

5. Repeat two to three times.

Stretches for the Upper Extremity

This chapter covers the muscles of the shoulder, arm, and wrist. The shoulder has the greatest range of motion of any joint in the body. We'll look at the four muscles of the rotator cuff, other shoulder stabilizers, muscles affecting motion about the shoulder, and the muscles that move the forearm and wrist.

Shoulder Stabilizers

The muscles that attach to and around the shoulder and shoulder blade provide stabilizing forces as well as active motion at the shoulder.

Anatomy: Rotator Cuff

The tendons of four muscles form the rotator cuff. They are the subscapularis, infraspinatus, teres minor, and supraspinatus. They are also referred to as the SITS muscles, a mnemonic device for remembering their names. These muscles, the prime movers of the arm at the shoulder, also stabilize the humerus in the glenoid fossa of the scapula during movement.

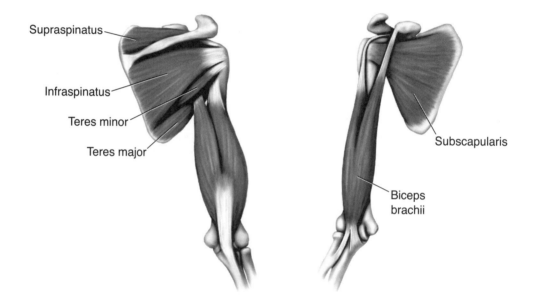

Supraspinatus

Infraspinatus

Teres minor

Teres major

Subscapularis

Biceps brachii

Muscle	Origin	Insertion	Action
ROTATOR CUFF MUSCLES			
Supraspinatus	Supraspinous fossa of scapula	Greater tubercle of humerus (superior facet)	Stabilizes head of humerus in glenoid fossa Initiates abduction
Infraspinatus	Infraspinous fossa of scapula	Greater tubercle of humerus (middle facet)	Lateral rotation of humerus
Teres minor	Upper axillary border of scapula	Greater tubercle of humerus (inferior facet)	Lateral rotation of humerus
Subscapularis	Subscapularis fossa of scapula	Lesser tubercle of humerus	Medial rotation of humerus

Anatomy: Scapular Stabilizers and Movers

We also include in this section a few muscles that stabilize and influence the motion of the shoulder blade. They are the serratus anterior, rhomboids, middle trapezius, and pectoralis minor.

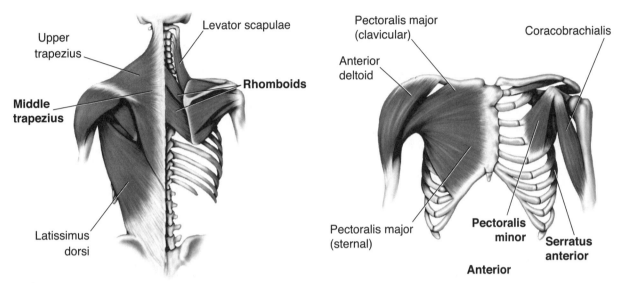

Muscle	Origin	Insertion	Action
SCAPULAR STABILIZERS AND MOVERS			
Rhomboid minor	Spinous processes of C7 and T1	Medial border of the scapula, at the root of the spine	Adducts, elevates, and downwardly rotates the scapula Helps stabilize the scapula during arm movements
Rhomboid major	Spinous processes of T2 through T5	Medial border of the scapula, from its spine to its inferior angle	Adducts, elevates, and downwardly rotates the scapula Helps stabilize the scapula during arm movements
Serratus anterior	A series of slips from the lateral aspect of the upper eight ribs and fascia The lower slips interdigitate with external obliques	The medial aspect of the costal surface of the scapula The upper slip attaches to the superior angle, the second through fourth slips attach along the medial border, and the lower four slips converge at the inferior angle	Protracts and laterally rotates the scapula
Middle trapezius	Spinous processes of C7 through T12 vertebrae	Spine of the scapula	Retracts the scapula
Pectoralis minor	Outer surface of the third, fourth, and fifth ribs, near the costochondral junctions	Medial border and superior surface at the tip of the coracoid process	Stabilizes the scapula by drawing it anteriorly and superiorly against the thoracic wall

SHOULDER STABILIZERS

Although the rhomboids often are tender to palpation, they are commonly overstretched rather than hypertonic. This overstretched condition is likely in people with rounded shoulders, in whom the pectoralis muscles draw the shoulders forward. In such a situation, stretching the pectorals and strengthening the rhomboids would be indicated. Refer to our discussion of this in chapter 1.

Functional Assessment: Shoulder Complex

Active movements can be used to evaluate the entire shoulder complex (humerus, clavicle, scapula) for freedom of movement and for pain. Restriction in range may be caused by hypertrophy or hypertonicity of the muscles or by pain.

Normal ranges of shoulder motion (figure 5.1):

Flexion = 180 degrees

Extension = 60 degrees

Adduction = 45 degrees

Abduction = 180 degrees

Internal rotation = 90 degrees

External rotation = 50 degrees

Horizontal adduction = 130 degrees

Horizontal abduction = 30 degrees

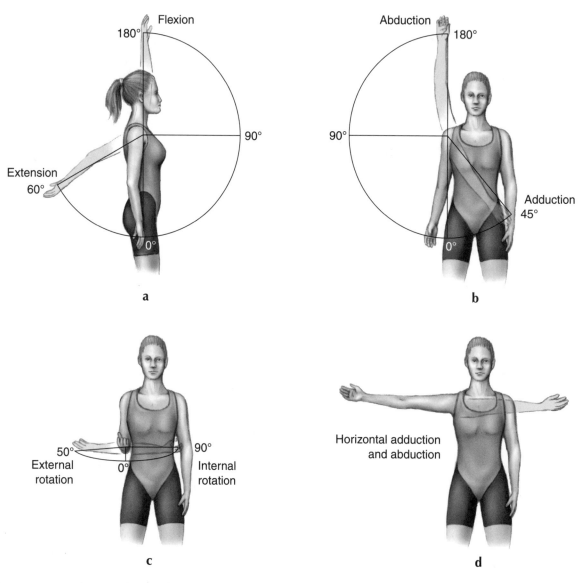

Figure 5.1 **Normal ranges of motion for the shoulder.**

Subscapularis Stretch, Supine, With a Partner

This stretch is used to improve external rotation of the humerus.

1. The stretcher is supine with her shoulder abducted to 90 degrees and her elbow flexed to 90 degrees. Her arm is externally rotated as far as possible, and her upper arm is resting completely on the table to avoid recruiting extra muscles. This lengthens the subscapularis to its pain-free end of range.

2. Offer resistance to the isometric contraction (no movement) of the subscapularis by placing one hand under the stretcher's elbow and the other hand over her wrist (figure 5.2).

3. Ask the stretcher to focus just on rotating her arm as you direct her to begin slowly to attempt to internally rotate her humerus, isometrically contracting the subscapularis for 6 seconds. ("Try to push your wrist toward the ceiling.")

4. After the isometric push, the stretcher relaxes and inhales deeply. During this time, maintain the arm in the starting position.

5. As she exhales, the stretcher contracts the infraspinatus to externally rotate the humerus farther, deepening the subscapularis stretch.

6. Repeat two to three times.

Subscapularis Self-Stretch, Standing at an Exercise Rack

1. An easy stretch for the subscapularis can be done at an exercise rack or in a doorway. Stand with your arm at your side, the elbow flexed to 90 degrees, and the humerus externally rotated as far as possible. It's helpful to think of the arm as a gate that swings back and forth (figure 5.3).

2. Use the doorjamb (or any fixed upright object) to resist your attempt to swing the gate closed (the arm pushes toward the stomach). Push for 6 seconds, isometrically contracting the subscapularis.

3. Stretch by "swinging the gate open" more.

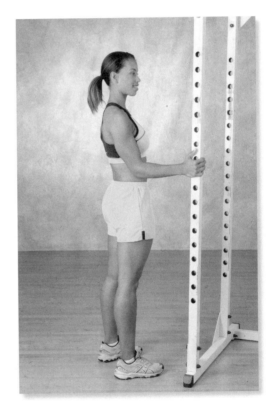

Figure 5.3 **Subscapularis self-stretch.**

Infraspinatus and Teres Minor Stretch, Prone, With a Partner

This stretch is used to improve internal rotation of the humerus.

1. The stretcher lies prone with her shoulder abducted to 90 degrees and her elbow flexed to 90 degrees. Her arm is internally rotated as

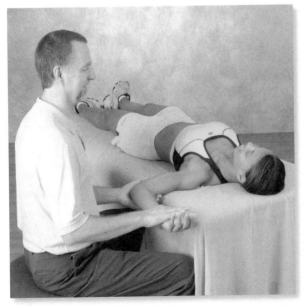

Figure 5.2 **Initiation of subscapularis stretch. The shoulder and elbow are both at 90 degrees, and the upper arm rests on the table.**

SHOULDER STABILIZERS

far as possible, and her upper arm is resting completely on the table to help avoid recruiting extra muscles. (The prone position helps prevent her shoulder from rolling forward, which would give a false impression of the range of internal rotation.) This position lengthens the infraspinatus to its pain-free end of range.

2. Offer resistance to the isometric contraction of the infraspinatus by placing one hand over the stretcher's elbow and the other hand under her wrist (figure 5.4).

3. Ask the stretcher to focus just on rotating her arm as you direct her to begin slowly to attempt to externally rotate her humerus, isometrically contracting the infraspinatus for 6 seconds. ("Try to push your wrist toward the floor.")

4. After the isometric push, the stretcher relaxes and inhales deeply. During this time, maintain the arm in the starting position.

5. As she exhales, the stretcher contracts the subscapularis to internally rotate the humerus farther, deepening the infraspinatus stretch.

6. Repeat two to three times.

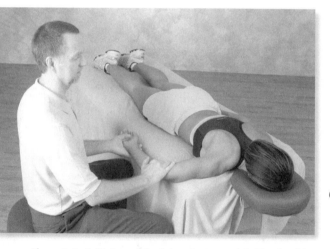

Figure 5.4 Initiation of the infraspinatus stretch. The shoulder and elbow are both at 90 degrees, and the upper arm rests on the table.

Infraspinatus and Teres Minor Self-Stretch, Standing

1. The infraspinatus can be a difficult muscle to self-stretch, but here is one option. Assume a "hammerlock" position—that is, with your left arm behind your back and your elbow flexed to approximately 90 degrees. Stand with your back to a door that is closed securely, and

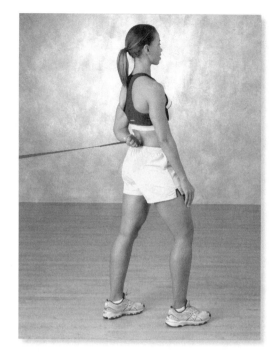

Figure 5.5 Infraspinatus self-stretch.

grasp the doorknob with your left hand. You may also attach a stretching strap to a piece of equipment (figure 5.5).

2. Holding the strap, try to push your forearm against your back, isometrically contracting the infraspinatus for 6 seconds.

3. Following the isometric contraction, pull your forearm farther away from your back as you take a step or two away from the piece of equipment, still holding on to the strap. This stretches the infraspinatus.

Serratus Anterior Stretch, Prone, With a Partner

This stretch is used to help reduce hypertonicity in the serratus anterior and to contribute to normal positioning of the scapula on the rib cage.

1. The stretcher is prone on the table with her arms resting at her sides. When her arm rests on the table, it's easier to move the shoulder blade. Stand at the head of the table and place the pads of your fingers (not the tips) against the lateral border of the right scapula. Direct the stretcher to pull her scapula toward her spine (retraction) as you assist. You may need to add some passive stretch to reach the soft tissue barrier for serratus. This lengthens the serratus anterior to its end range (figure 5.6).

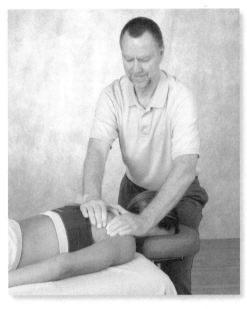

Figure 5.6   **Initiation of serratus anterior stretch.**

2. From this starting position, direct the stretcher to push her shoulder blade into your fingers (protraction), isometrically contracting the serratus anterior for 6 seconds.

3. After the isometric push, the stretcher relaxes and breathes, and as she exhales, uses her rhomboids to pull her shoulder blade closer to her spine as you assist. This deepens the stretch on serratus anterior.

4. Repeat two to three times.

Serratus Anterior Self-Stretch

1. Stand in a doorway or next to a fixed vertical object that you can safely push against. Place your left hand against the wall at about shoulder height. First use your back muscles (rhomboids) to pull your left shoulder blade closer to your spine; then lean your torso forward and twist to the right to push your left arm behind you. This will move the shoulder blade more toward the spine and increase the stretch on serratus anterior (figure 5.7).

2. From this starting position, push your left arm against the wall, but don't allow any movement. Hold this isometric contraction of serratus anterior for 6 seconds. Then relax and breathe.

3. As you exhale, to deepen the stretch of serratus anterior, pull your shoulder blade closer to your spine by leaning your torso forward and twisting to the left.

4. Repeat two to three times.

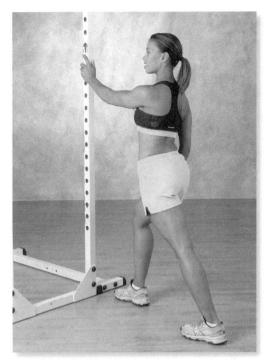

Figure 5.7   **Serratus anterior self-stretch.**

Rhomboids and Middle Trapezius Stretch, With a Partner, Supine

This stretch is used to improve scapular protraction (movement of the scapula away from the midline).

1. The stretcher is supine. With her left arm flexed at the elbow, she brings her humerus across her chest as far as possible. She may assist this motion by pulling with her right hand. She does not roll her torso up to the right, but keeps at least part of her scapula in contact with the table. This lengthens the left rhomboids to their end range.

2. Stand facing her left side. Reach under her back so that your hands are in firm contact with the body of the left scapula and so that your right fingers grasp its medial border (figure 5.8. p. 88). Ask the stretcher to begin slowly to try to pull her scapula toward her spine. You provide matching resistance for this 6-second isometric contraction, being sure that the client is breathing normally throughout. Be sure she engages her rhomboids and is not just pushing from her arm.

3. After the isometric push, the stretcher relaxes and breathes in. As she relaxes, maintain the scapula and arm in the starting position.

SHOULDER STABILIZERS

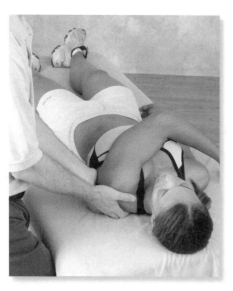

Figure 5.8 Initiation of supine rhomboids and middle trapezius stretch.

4. As she exhales, ask her to pull her arm farther across her chest, protracting the scapula farther away from the spine and increasing the rhomboid stretch.

5. Repeat two to three times.

Rhomboids and Middle Trapezius Stretch, With a Partner, Side-Lying

This stretch is used to improve scapular protraction (movement of the scapula away from the midline).

1. The stretcher lies on her right side, with her head resting on her right arm to help stabilize her torso. She reaches her left arm over the side of the table, focusing on moving her scapula away from her spine, to lengthen the rhomboids and middle trapezius to their end range.

2. Stand behind the stretcher and place your hands on her scapula so that your flat thumbs can palpate the medial border (figure 5.9). Direct the stretcher to begin slowly to try to pull her scapula back toward her spine, isometrically contracting her rhomboids and middle trapezius for 6 seconds. During this time, the focus is on the scapula. Her left arm should be relaxed.

3. After the isometric push, the stretcher relaxes and inhales. As she exhales, she reaches farther over the edge of the table to deepen the stretch on the rhomboids and middle trapezius.

4. Repeat two to three times.

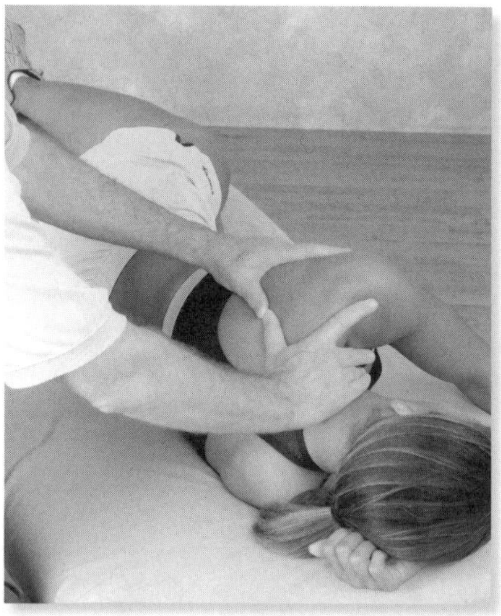

Figure 5.9 Initiation of side-lying rhomboids and middle trapezius stretch.

Rhomboids and Middle Trapezius Self-Stretch, Sitting

1. Flex your arm and shoulder to 90 degrees and bring your arm across your chest. This pulls your scapula away from your spine and stretches your rhomboids. Use your other hand to hold at your elbow, stabilizing your arm.

2. Try to bring your scapula toward your spine, isometrically contracting your rhomboids for 6 seconds.

3. After the isometric contraction, stretch the rhomboids by bringing your arm farther across your chest (figure 5.10).

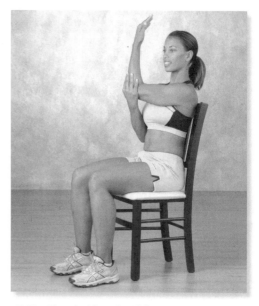

Figure 5.10 Rhomboids and middle trapezius self-stretch.

Pectoralis Minor Stretch, Supine, With a Partner

This stretch is for reducing hypertonicity in the pectoralis minor and to help normalize the position of the scapula on the rib cage.

1. The stretcher lies supine on the table. Stand at her left side and hold her left hand in your left hand, allowing her upper arm to rest at her side, on the table. This position keeps her arm from bouncing around. Place the fleshy part of your right palm on her anterior shoulder. Direct the stretcher to pull her shoulder toward the table and her shoulder blade down her back toward her feet. ("Put your shoulder blade in your back pocket.") You may assist this motion passively. This lengthens the pectoralis minor to its end range (figure 5.11).

2. Direct the stretcher to start slowly and try to roll her shoulder up into your right hand, isometrically contracting pectoralis minor for 6 seconds.

3. After the isometric push, the stretcher relaxes and breathes in. As she exhales, ask the stretcher to once again pull her shoulder

toward the table and her shoulder blade down her back as you gently assist. This deepens the stretch on pectoralis minor.

4. Repeat two to three times.

Pectoralis Minor Self-Stretch, Standing

1. Stand with your hands clasped behind your back. Stand at attention and try to pull your shoulder blades down your back. This position puts the pectoralis minor on a stretch.

2. Place the front of your right shoulder against a doorjamb or other fixed upright, and begin slowly to try to roll your shoulder forward (figure 5.12).

3. Hold this isometric contraction for 6 seconds, then relax, breathe, and try to once again pull your shoulders back and down, stretching the pectoralis minor.

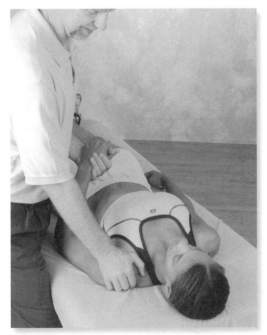

Figure 5.11 Initiation of pectoralis minor stretch.

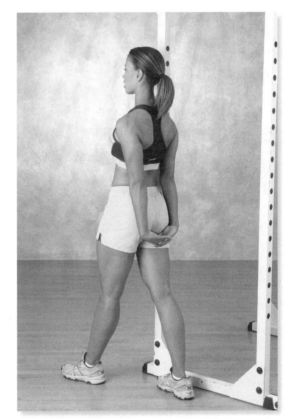

Figure 5.12 Pectoralis minor self-stretch.

SHOULDER STABILIZERS

Pectoralis Major, Biceps, Triceps

We'll look at three additional muscles that affect the shoulder: the pectoralis major, the biceps brachii, and the triceps.

Anatomy

Pectoralis major is a broad, powerful muscle that gives shape to the chest and is a strong mover of the arm. It is divided into two sections: the clavicular head and the sternal head. Acting together, these help adduct, horizontally adduct, and medially rotate the humerus. The clavicular head, acting alone, assists flexion of the humerus. The sternal head, acting alone, extends the humerus from a flexed position.

The biceps brachii is a two-headed, two-joint muscle. It crosses both the shoulder and the elbow and affects both. Primarily, biceps brachii assists flexion of the shoulder, flexion of the elbow, and supination of the forearm.

The triceps is a three-headed, two-joint muscle. It crosses both the shoulder and the elbow and acts on both. Its primary action is extension of the elbow. The long head assists extension of the humerus.

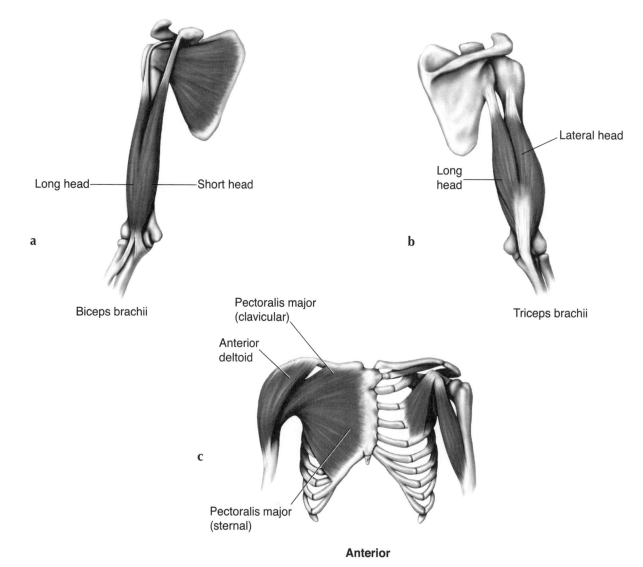

Long head — Short head

a

Biceps brachii

Lateral head

Long head

b

Triceps brachii

Pectoralis major (clavicular)

Anterior deltoid

c

Pectoralis major (sternal)

Anterior

Muscle	Origin	Insertion	Action
PECTORALIS, BICEPS, AND TRICEPS			
Pectoralis major	Clavicular head: medial half of anterior aspect of clavicle Sternal head: sternum and cartilage of the six upper ribs	Lateral lip of bicipital groove of the humerus	Both heads: adduction, horizontal adduction, and medial rotation of the humerus Clavicular head: flexion of humerus Sternal head: extension of humerus from a flexed position
Biceps brachii	Long head: tubercle on superior aspect of glenoid cavity Short head: coracoid process	Radial tuberosity and bicipital aponeurosis	Elbow and shoulder flexion Supination of forearm Long head assists abduction Short head assists adduction Helps stabilize humerus in glenoid fossa during heavy lifting or carrying
Triceps brachii	Long head: infraglenoid tubercle of scapula Lateral head: posterolateral surface of proximal humerus Medial head: lower two-thirds of posteromedial humerus	Olecranon process of ulna	Extension of elbow Long head only: extension of humerus

Functional Assessment

Normal range of motion at the elbow (figure 5.13):

Flexion = 150 degrees

Extension = 0 degrees

Elbow flexion may be limited by the muscle mass of the anterior arm or by a hypertonic triceps. Generally, the stretcher should be able to touch the front of her shoulder.

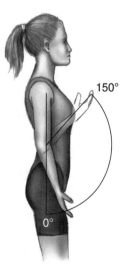

Figure 5.13 **Normal flexion-extension of the elbow.**

PECTORALIS MAJOR, BICEPS, TRICEPS

Pectoralis Major Stretch, Prone, With a Partner

Stretching the pectoralis major can improve range of motion in horizontal abduction, flexion, extension, and external rotation of the humerus, depending on which fibers of the muscle are emphasized during the stretch. *Note:* By changing the angle of abduction of the arm, you can emphasize different fibers of the pectoralis major. Less abduction (45 degrees) focuses on the clavicular head; more abduction (135 degrees) focuses more on the lower fibers of the sternocostal head.

1. The stretcher is prone, with her face resting in the face cradle, or her head turned to one side if no face cradle is available. Her right arm is abducted to 90 degrees and externally rotated, with the elbow bent to 90 degrees. Her upper arm rests on the table. Stand at the right side of the table and ask the stretcher to lift her right arm toward the ceiling as high as possible, keeping the forearm horizontal. As she lifts, make sure she does not lift her sternum off the table, which would indicate that she is rotating her trunk. This starting position lengthens the right pectoralis major to its pain-free end range.

2. Support the stretcher's right arm from the elbow to the hand using your right forearm and hand (figure 5.14). Ask the stretcher to begin slowly to attempt to bring her arm down and across her chest, leading with the elbow, isometrically contracting the pectoralis major for 6 seconds. During the isometric contraction of the pectoralis major, the rhomboids should be relaxed.

3. After the isometric push, the stretcher relaxes and breathes in. During this time, maintain the arm in the starting position.

4. As she exhales, ask the stretcher to lift her arm higher, keeping the forearm horizontal and her sternum on the table to prevent trunk rotation.

5. Repeat two to three times. Remember that changing the angle of abduction of the arm emphasizes different fibers of the pectoralis major.

Pectoralis Major Self-Stretch, at an Exercise Rack

You can perform self-stretching of the pectoralis using an exercise rack, a doorway, or any other vertical column to provide resistance during the isometric phase. Raise your arm higher or lower to stretch different parts of the pectoralis. *Note:* Raising your arm higher against the vertical column will emphasize the pectoralis fibers that attach to the sternum. Having your arm lower on the vertical column will emphasize the fibers that attach to the collarbone.

1. Stand at an exercise rack and place your forearm against it. Be aware of your posture and use a wide front-to-back lunge stance, keeping your back lengthened and not arched. Using your upper back muscles, pull your arm backward, away from the vertical column as far as you can; then take a step or two forward until your forearm is once again placed against the vertical column. This is your starting position (figure 5.15).

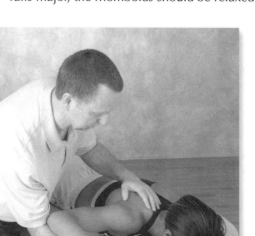

Figure 5.14 Initiation of the pectoralis major stretch. Be sure that the stretcher does not lift the sternum off the table.

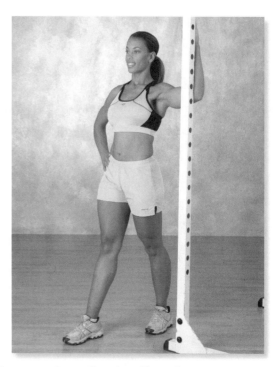

Figure 5.15 Pectoralis major self-stretch.

2. Start slowly and push with moderate effort against the column, isometrically contracting the pectoralis major. Your arm is not moving, just pushing. Breathe normally. Hold the push for 6 seconds, then relax.

3. Take another breath, and as you exhale, use your upper back muscles to pull your arm backward, away from the column, as far as you can. This further stretches the pectoralis major.

4. Repeat two to three times.

Biceps Brachii Stretch, Supine, With a Partner

This stretch is for improving the range of elbow and shoulder extension.

1. The stretcher lies supine with her left shoulder at the edge of the table to ensure full range of motion of the shoulder. Her left elbow is straight, and her shoulder is extended as far as possible. Her forearm is in neutral, neither supinated nor pronated (the palm faces inward). This position lengthens the bicep to its end range.

2. Offer resistance to the isometric contraction of the biceps by placing your right hand against the stretcher's left forearm. Use your left hand to stabilize her shoulder (figure 5.16).

3. Direct the stretcher to begin slowly to attempt to flex her left shoulder and elbow and supi-

nate her forearm, isometrically contracting the biceps brachii for 6 seconds. ("Try to turn your forearm, bend your elbow, and lift your arm toward the ceiling.")

4. After the isometric push, the stretcher relaxes and inhales deeply. During this time, the arm may drop toward the floor or be maintained in the starting position.

5. As she exhales, the stretcher contracts the triceps to extend the arm farther, deepening the biceps stretch.

6. Repeat two to three times.

Biceps Brachii Self-Stretch

The biceps brachii can be an awkward muscle to self-stretch, but it can be done.

1. Find a horizontal surface, like a railing, a dance barre, or the back of a chair. You can also use the doorknob on a closed door. Stand (or kneel) with your arm straight, palm facing inward, and extend your arm behind you as far as you can, keeping your torso upright. Rest your forearm on the horizontal object or grasp the doorknob.

2. From this starting position, try to push your hand toward the floor (flexion of the shoulder and elbow), isometrically contracting the biceps for 6 seconds.

3. After the isometric phase, extend your arm back farther. You may need to kneel down to properly position yourself for this stretch (figure 5.17).

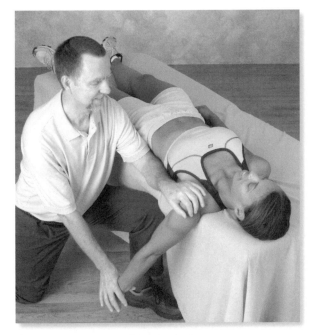

Figure 5.16   Initiation of biceps stretch.

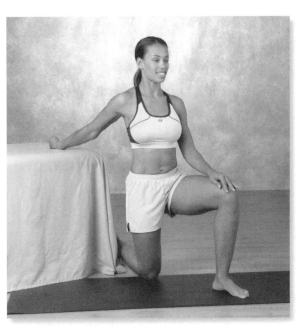

Figure 5.17   Biceps self-stretch.

PECTORALIS MAJOR, BICEPS, TRICEPS

Triceps Stretch, Prone, With a Partner

This stretch is used to improve flexion at the shoulder with the elbow bent.

1. The stretcher is prone, with her head resting in the face cradle or turned to the side. She flexes her right shoulder and elbow and reaches toward her shoulder blade, keeping her arm as close to her ear as possible (figure 5.18). The flat part of the elbow (posterior humerus) points toward the floor, not out to the side. This lengthens the triceps to their end range.

2. Place your hand against the stretcher's posterior elbow and ask her to begin to push slowly against you, attempting to bring her elbow toward the floor, isometrically contracting the triceps for 6 seconds.

3. After the isometric push, the stretcher relaxes and breathes in. During this time, maintain the arm in the starting position.

4. As she exhales, ask the stretcher to reach farther down her back, keeping her arm close to her ear, deepening the triceps stretch.

5. Repeat the sequence two to three more times.

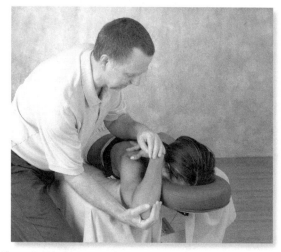

Figure 5.18   **Initiation of triceps stretch.**

Triceps Self-Stretch

1. Stand tall, keeping your back and neck lengthened. This stretch can also be done sitting.

2. Flex your right shoulder and elbow to try to touch your right shoulder blade. Keep your arm as close to your ear as possible, with the flat part of the elbow pointing toward the front, not out to the side. This lengthens the triceps to its end range.

3. You provide isometric resistance for this stretch by using your other arm and hand as shown in the photo (figure 5.19). Be sure to keep your neck lengthened as you reach around. Hold the contraction for 6 seconds, breathing normally.

4. After the isometric push, relax, take a deep breath in, and as you exhale, stretch by reaching farther down your back. Be sure to maintain length in the spine (low back and neck) during this stretch to achieve the best results.

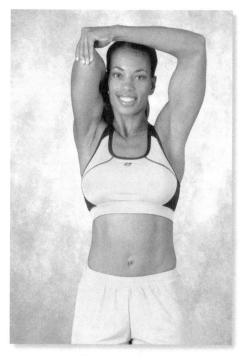

Figure 5.19   **Triceps self-stretch. Avoid arching your low back.**

Muscles of the Wrist and Hand

Anatomy: Wrist Flexors and Extensors

Baseball players, racquetball players, musicians, grocery clerks, and typists commonly have hypertonic wrist and forearm muscles. Maintaining good range of motion at the wrist can help reduce the risk of overuse tendinitis or repetitive stress injuries like carpal tunnel syndrome.

Limited range of motion at the wrist is uncommon unless the wrist has been immobilized for some reason. Because the wrist muscles are used extensively in daily activity, even "leg sport" athletes will appreciate stretching these muscles.

▌ *Wrist flexors*—Three primary muscles act to flex the wrist: flexor carpi radialis, flexor carpi ulnaris, and palmaris longus. Their common origin on the medial epicondyle is the site of "golfer's elbow," an overuse tendinitis.

▌ *Wrist extensors*—Like the flexors of the wrist, three primary muscles extend the wrist: extensor carpi radialis longus, extensor carpi radialis brevis, and extensor carpi ulnaris. Their common origin on the lateral epicondyle is the primary site of "tennis elbow," an overuse tendinitis common in racket sports.

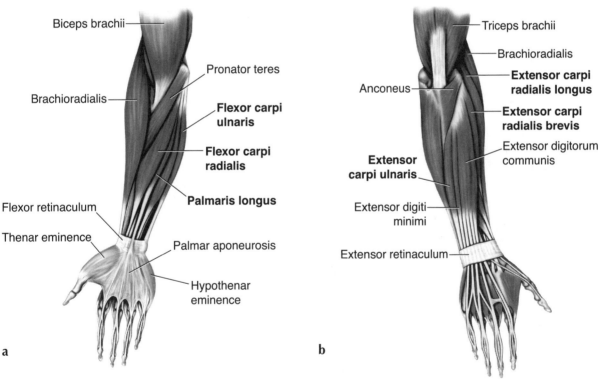

a

b

Muscle	Origin	Insertion	Action
WRIST FLEXORS			
Flexor carpi radialis	Medial epicondyle of humerus	Base of second and third metacarpals	Flexion and abduction of wrist
Flexor carpi ulnaris	Medial epicondyle of humerus and proximal posterior ulna	Pisiform, hamate, and base of fifth metacarpal	Flexion and adduction of wrist
Palmaris longus (sometimes absent)	Medial epicondyle of humerus	Palmar aponeurosis	Assists flexion of wrist
WRIST EXTENSORS			
Extensor carpi radialis longus	Lateral epicondyle and lateral supracondylar ridge of humerus	Base of second metacarpal	Extension and abduction of wrist
Extensor carpi radialis brevis	Lateral epicondyle of humerus	Base of third metacarpal	Extension of wrist
Extensor carpi ulnaris	Lateral epicondyle of humerus and proximal posterior ulna	Base of fifth metacarpal	Extension and adduction of wrist

Anatomy: Forearm Pronators and Supinator

The pronators and supinator are often overlooked as sources of pain.

■ *Forearm pronators*—Pronator teres dysfunction can mimic the pain of medial epicondylitis ("golfer's elbow"); and trigger points in this muscle refer to the radial side of the wrist, prompting some people to self-diagnose carpal tunnel syndrome. Pronator teres syndrome is caused by compression of the median nerve and is characterized by numbness in the median nerve distribution, aching deep in the forearm, and hand weakness. When both pronators are hypertonic, the forearms at rest tend to be pronated.

■ *Forearm supinator*—The supinator can mimic the pain of lateral epicondylitis ("tennis elbow"). The supinator can be injured as a result of excessive eccentric stress placed upon it, especially during activities when the elbow is held straight, as in performing the backhand in tennis, carrying a heavy suitcase, or even holding the leash while walking the dog. The radial nerve passes between the deep and the superficial parts of the supinator, and nerve entrapment is usually characterized by weakness, rather than pain.

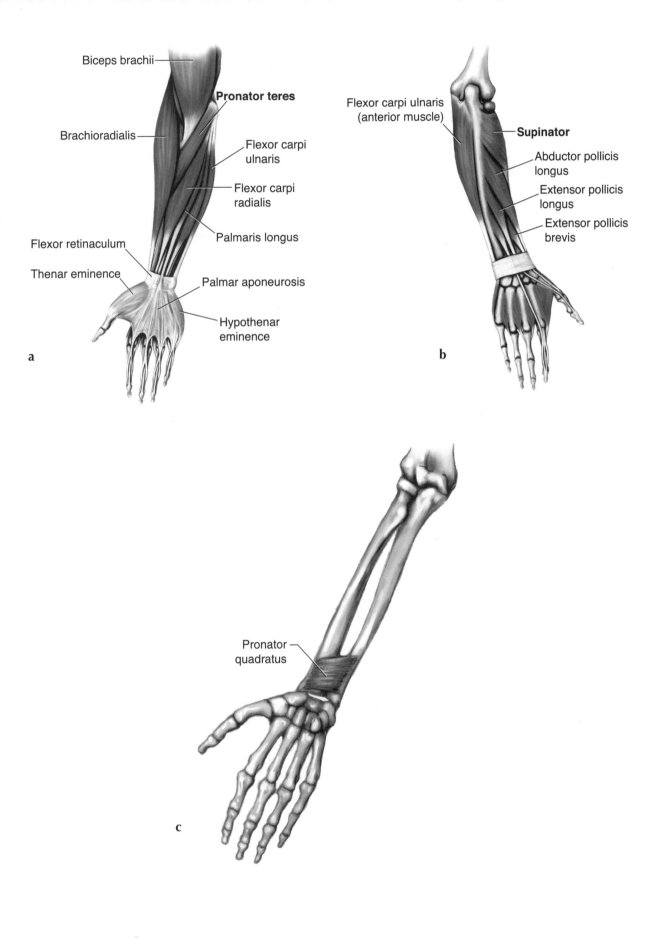

Biceps brachii

Pronator teres

Brachioradialis

Flexor carpi ulnaris

Flexor carpi radialis

Palmaris longus

Flexor retinaculum

Thenar eminence

Palmar aponeurosis

Hypothenar eminence

a

Flexor carpi ulnaris (anterior muscle)

Supinator

Abductor pollicis longus

Extensor pollicis longus

Extensor pollicis brevis

b

Pronator quadratus

c

MUSCLES OF THE WRIST AND HAND

MUSCLES OF THE WRIST AND HAND

Muscle	Origin	Insertion	Action
PRONATORS AND SUPINATOR OF FOREARM			
Pronator quadratus	Anterior aspect of the distal one-fourth of the ulna	Anterior aspect of the distal one-fourth of the radius	Principal pronator of the forearm
Pronator teres	Medial aspect of the coronoid process of the ulna and the medial epicondyle of the humerus	Halfway along the lateral surface of the radius	Pronation of the forearm (secondary to pronator quadratus) and weak elbow flexion
Supinator	Lateral epicondyle of the humerus, radial collateral and annular ligaments of the elbow, the supinator crest and fossa of the ulna	Lateral aspect of the proximal third of the radius	Supination of the forearm when the elbow is extended Assists flexion when the elbow is already bent and forearm supinated
Biceps brachii	Long head: tubercle on superior aspect of glenoid cavity Short head: coracoid process	Radial tuberosity and bicipital aponeurosis	Elbow and shoulder flexion Supination of forearm Long head assists abduction Short head assists adduction Helps stabilize humerus in glenoid fossa during heavy lifting or carrying

Functional Assessment

Normal range of motion, measured from the wrist in neutral (figure 5.20):

Flexion = 80 degrees
Extension = 70 degrees
Ulnar deviation (adduction) = 30 degrees

Radial deviation (abduction) = 20 degrees
Pronation = 90 degrees
Supination = 90 degrees

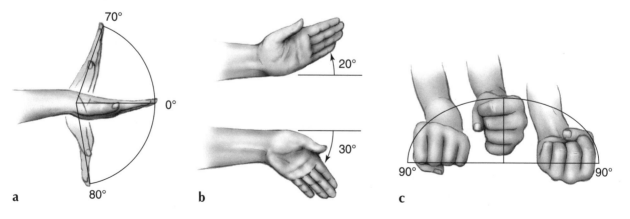

a   b   c

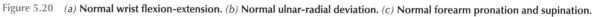

Figure 5.20   *(a)* **Normal wrist flexion-extension.** *(b)* **Normal ulnar-radial deviation.** *(c)* **Normal forearm pronation and supination.**

Wrist and Finger Flexors Stretch, Supine, With a Partner

This stretch is used for increasing extension at the wrist.

1. The stretcher is supine, with his right elbow straight, arm resting on the table if possible, and his wrist and fingers extended as far as possible. Make sure the table is not blocking full extension of the wrist. This lengthens the right wrist (and finger) flexors to their pain-free end range.

2. Place the palm and fingers of your left hand over the palm and fingers of the stretcher's right hand, matching thumb to thumb and finger to finger. Your other hand stabilizes the stretcher's wrist and forearm (figure 5.21).

3. Direct the stretcher to start slowly to try to flex his wrist and fingers (including the thumb), isometrically contracting the flexors for 6 seconds.

4. After the isometric push, the stretcher relaxes and breathes in. During this time, maintain his wrist and fingers in the starting position.

5. As he exhales, the stretcher contracts the wrist and finger extensors, deepening the wrist flexor stretch. You may gently assist in deepening the stretch by pushing on the stretcher's fingers.

6. Repeat two to three times.

Wrist and Finger Flexors Self-Stretch, Sitting

1. To stretch the wrist flexors, sit comfortably with your right arm out in front of you, elbow straight, and wrist and fingers extended as far as possible. This lengthens the right wrist (and finger) flexors to their pain-free end range.

2. Place the palm and fingers of your left hand over the palm and fingers of your right hand (figure 5.22). Start slowly to try to flex the wrist and fingers (including the thumb) against the resistance of your left hand, isometrically contracting the right wrist flexors for 6 seconds.

3. After the isometric push, relax and breathe in, maintaining the wrist and fingers in the starting position. As you exhale, contract the right wrist and finger extensors, deepening the wrist flexor stretch. You may gently assist in deepening the stretch by pushing on your fingers.

4. Repeat two to three times.

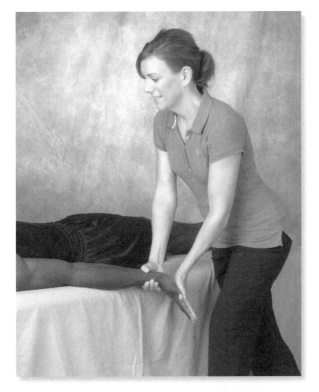

Figure 5.21 **Initiation of the wrist and finger flexors stretch.**

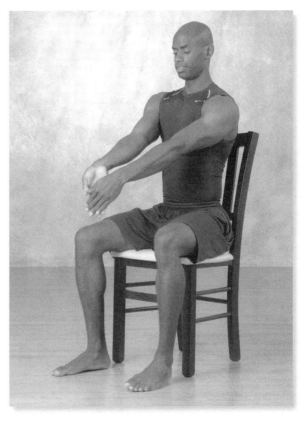

Figure 5.22 **Wrist and finger flexors self-stretch.**

MUSCLES OF THE WRIST AND HAND

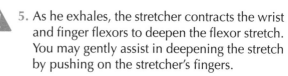

Wrist and Finger Extensors Stretch, Supine, With a Partner

This stretch is used for increasing wrist and finger flexion.

1. The stretcher is supine, with his right elbow straight, arm resting on the table, and his wrist and fingers flexed as far as possible. Be sure the table is not blocking the full flexion of his wrist. This will lengthen the right wrist (and finger) extensors to their pain-free end range. (The stretcher should fully flex his wrist first, and then curl his fingers as far as possible. Curling the fingers first will limit his wrist flexion and our primary goal is to maximize wrist flexion.

2. Wrap your right hand over the stretcher's fist, matching thumb to thumb and finger to finger. Your other hand stabilizes the stretcher's wrist and forearm (figure 5.23).

3. Direct the stretcher to start slowly to try to extend the wrist and fingers (including the thumb), isometrically contracting the extensors for 6 seconds.

4. After the isometric push, the stretcher relaxes and breathes in. During this time, maintain his wrist and fingers in the starting position.

5. As he exhales, the stretcher contracts the wrist and finger flexors to deepen the flexor stretch. You may gently assist in deepening the stretch by pushing on the stretcher's fingers.

6. Repeat two to three times.

Wrist and Finger Extensors Self-Stretch, Sitting

1. To stretch the wrist extensors, sit comfortably with your right arm out in front of you, elbow straight, and wrist and fingers flexed as far as possible. This lengthens the right wrist (and finger) extensors to their pain-free end range. Fully flex your wrist first, then curl your fingers as far as possible. Curling the fingers first will limit your wrist flexion and your primary goal is to maximize wrist flexion.

2. Wrap your left hand around your right to provide resistance, then start slowly to try to extend your wrist and fingers (including the thumb), isometrically contracting the extensors for 6 seconds (figure 5.24).

3. After the isometric push, relax and breathe in, maintaining your wrist and fingers in the starting position. As you exhale, contract the right wrist and finger flexors, deepening the stretch on the extensors.

4. Repeat two to three times.

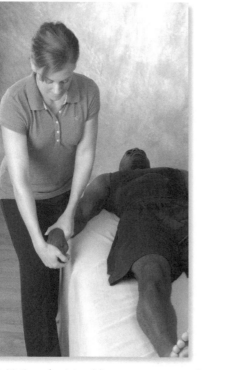

Figure 5.23 Initiation of wrist and finger extensors stretch.

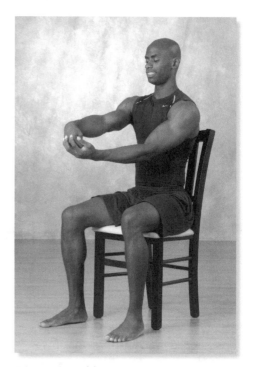

Figure 5.24 Wrist and finger extensors self-stretch.

MUSCLES OF THE WRIST AND HAND

Forearm Supinator Stretch, Supine, With a Partner

This stretch is used for increasing pronation of the forearm.

1. The stretcher is supine with his right upper arm resting at his side, elbow flexed to about 90 degrees, so it's easy for you to stand at his side and grasp the wrist. The stretcher pronates his right forearm and hand (palm turns down) as far as possible. This lengthens the supinator to its pain-free end range.

2. Support the forearm with one hand, and the wrist and hand with the other, being careful to keep the wrist in neutral, neither flexed nor extended, to avoid undue stress on the joint (figure 5.25). Your grasp should span the wrist from proximal to distal to minimize any twisting stress on the joint.

3. Direct the stretcher to start slowly to try to supinate his forearm (turn his palm up), isometrically contracting the supinator for 6 seconds.

4. After the isometric push, the stretcher relaxes and breathes in. During this time, maintain his forearm in the starting position.

5. As he exhales, the stretcher contracts the pronators to deepen the supinator stretch.

6. Repeat two to three times.

Forearm Supinator Self-Stretch, Sitting

1. Sit comfortably, bend your left elbow, and rotate your left forearm to the right so that your palm faces down. This position stretches the supinator.

2. Wrap your right hand over your left so that the fingers of your right hand can hold on to the little-finger side of your left hand and wrist (figure 5.26).

3. From this starting position, begin slowly and try to rotate your forearm back to the left (supination), isometrically contracting your supinator for 6 seconds. After the contraction, relax and breathe in.

4. As you exhale, rotate your forearm more to the right to deepen the stretch on the supinator.

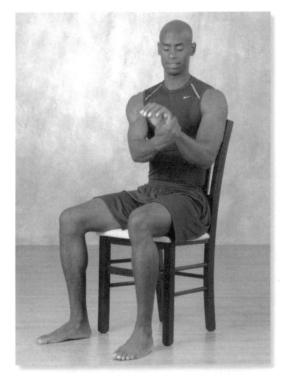

Figure 5.26 **Supinator self-stretch.**

Forearm Pronators Stretch, Supine, With a Partner

This stretch is used for improving range of motion in supination.

1. The stretcher is supine with his right upper arm resting at his side, elbow flexed to about 90 degrees, so it's easy for you to stand at his

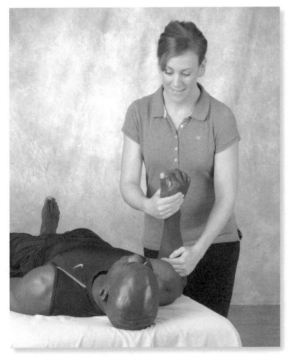

Figure 5.25 **Initiation of the supinator stretch.**

side and grasp the wrist. His right forearm is supinated as far as possible, stretching the pronators to their pain-free end range.

2. Stand facing the stretcher; support his forearm with your right hand, and with your left, grasp his hand and wrist. (Supporting the wrist in neutral helps prevent undue stress on the carpal bones, figure 5.27.) Your grasp should span the wrist from proximal to distal to minimize any twisting stress on the joint.

3. Direct the stretcher to start slowly to try to pronate his forearm (turn his palm down), isometrically contracting his pronators for 6 seconds.

4. After the isometric push, the stretcher relaxes and breathes in. During this time, maintain his forearm in the starting position.

5. As he exhales, the stretcher supinates to deepen the stretch of the pronators. You may gently assist in deepening the stretch by adding some passive supination.

6. Repeat two to three times.

Forearm Pronators Self-Stretch, Sitting

1. Sit comfortably, bend your left elbow, and rotate your left forearm to the left so that your palm faces up. This position stretches the pronators. Wrap your right hand under your left so that the fingers of your right hand can hold on to the thumb side of your left hand and wrist (figure 5.28).

2. From this starting position, begin slowly and try to rotate your forearm back to the left (pronation), isometrically contracting your pronators for 6 seconds. After the contraction, relax and breathe in.

3. As you exhale, contract your supinators by rotating your forearm more to the left to deepen the stretch on the pronators.

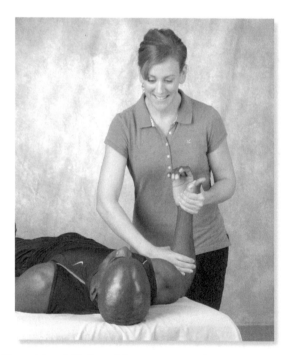

Figure 5.27 **Initiation of the pronator stretch.**

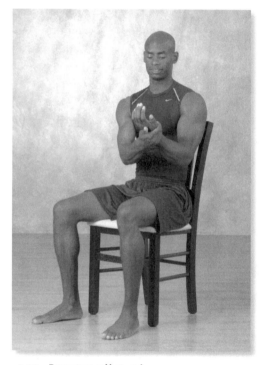

Figure 5.28 **Pronators self-stretch.**

Spiral–Diagonal Patterns for the Upper Extremity

The spiral–diagonal patterns for the arms are extremely useful for increasing range of motion in the shoulder girdle. They're also helpful in determining which muscles in a pattern of motion are weak or are not firing properly. These individual muscles can then be isolated for single-plane stretching or strengthening.

Working with the upper extremity can seem complicated because we have the option of working with the elbow bent or straight in the two patterns that involve adduction (flexion end of D1 and extension end of D2). Here we give the instructions assuming that the elbow remains straight. As you gain more experience, you can work with the elbow bent and add resisted elbow extension during the isometric phase.

Compared to the single-plane stretches, using the patterns requires more concentration from both the stretcher and you. Accordingly, we recommend that you illustrate what you want the stretcher to do by taking him through the pattern passively a few times before attempting to perform the stretch.

Remember that we use only the lengthened range of the pattern. Our goal is to improve range of motion into the lengthening direction. The stretch happens when the stretcher moves farther into the lengthened range after the isometric contraction.

Before proceeding with the exercises, you may find it useful to review, in chapter 3, the arm patterns on pages 19 through 22 as well as the discussion about the change in nomenclature from the previous edition on page 21.

Draw Sword Stretch (Flexion End of D2)

This stretch is for improving range of motion in flexion, abduction, and external rotation.

1. The stretcher lies supine, so that his joint line is just beyond the edge of the table. His left shoulder is flexed, abducted, and externally rotated as far as possible. His forearm is supinated, with the wrist and fingers in neutral. This is the starting position for the flexion end of D2 and lengthens the target muscles to their end range. These include the pectorals (sternal head), anterior deltoid, subscapularis, biceps brachii, pronator teres, latissimus dorsi, and teres major.

2. Support and stabilize the arm and wrist (figure 5.29). Remember, your hand contacts give the stretcher proprioceptive cues about which way to push or pull; your hand positions should match your verbal commands. Your grasp spans the wrist and hand and across the elbow to minimize stress on the joints.

3. Direct the stretcher to begin slowly to try to initiate the D2 extension pattern, first with internal rotation, then adduction, then extension. ("Begin by rotating, then try to reach down to touch your right hip.") The stretcher is not trying to bend his elbow.

4. After the isometric push, the stretcher relaxes and inhales deeply. As he relaxes, maintain the arm in the starting position.

5. As he exhales, the stretcher moves his arm farther into flexion, then into abduction, and then into external rotation and supination. Remember, we want a blend of all three directions to keep moving in a diagonal line. Support the arm but do not push to deepen the stretch.

6. Repeat two to three times.

Draw Sword Self-Stretch

1. Attach a stretching strap to a fixed object above and behind you. To use a cable and pulley machine at the gym, select the maximum weight so that you cannot lift it. Stand (or sit on a stability ball) so that you can reach your right arm up, out, and rotated as if you were holding a sword (or an Olympic torch!). Grab on to the stretching strap or the handle of the machine. Keep your torso from twisting by focusing on stretching from the shoulder joint. This is the start of the "draw sword" stretch (figure 5.30).

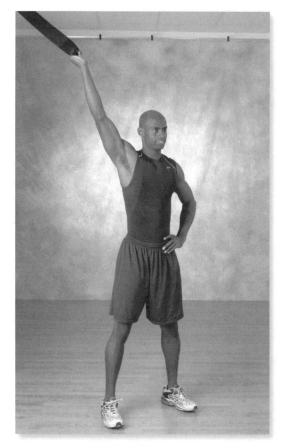

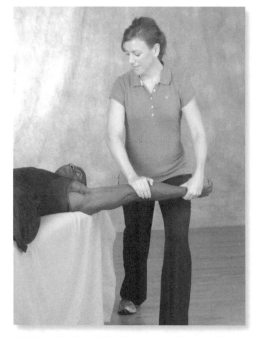

Figure 5.29 Initiation of the "draw sword" stretch (D2 pattern). The arm is flexed, abducted, and externally rotated.

Figure 5.30 "Draw sword" self-stretch.

2. Start slowly and rotate your arm, then pull down and across as if you were putting a sword back into its scabbard, or as if to touch your left hip. Use the stretching strap to resist this attempt at motion, and hold this isometric contraction for 6 seconds. Then relax and breathe.

3. As you exhale, reach up, out, and back; then turn your arm a little more to deepen the stretch on the target muscles. Focus on stretching out of the shoulder joint, and keep your back flat as you stretch. Take up any slack on the stretching strap or reposition yourself at the cable machine, and repeat the sequence two to three times.

Sheath Sword Stretch (Extension End of D2)

This stretch is used to improve range of motion in extension, adduction, and internal rotation. The stretch position is different from that in free-exercise practice. During free exercise, we stop at the front of the hip; but remember that the spiral pattern continues through the body to the end of available range in extension, adduction, and internal rotation. So the stretch begins with the arm behind the back.

1. The stretcher is prone, with his left shoulder extended, adducted, and internally rotated. The forearm is pronated, with the wrist and fingers in neutral. This starting position is a modified hammerlock. The stretcher keeps his elbow straight while adducting across the back as far as possible, with his thumb pointing away from his back. This position lengthens the target muscles to their end range. These include the anterior deltoid, coracobrachialis, pectorals, and biceps brachii.

2. Support and stabilize the arm and wrist (figure 5.31). Remember, your hand contacts give the stretcher proprioceptive cues about which way to push or pull; your hand positions should match your verbal commands. Your grasp spans the wrist and hand and across the elbow to minimize stress on the joints.

3. Direct the stretcher to begin slowly to try to initiate the D2 flexion pattern, first with external rotation, then abduction, then flexion. ("Begin by rotating, then push through and away from your body.")

4. After the isometric push, the stretcher relaxes and inhales deeply. As he relaxes, maintain the arm in the starting position.

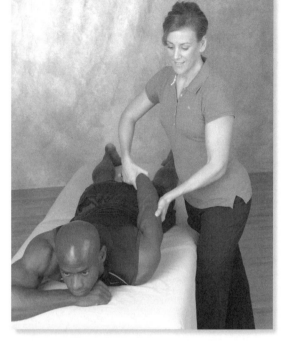

Figure 5.31 Initiation of the "sheath sword" stretch (D2 pattern). The arm is extended, adducted, and internally rotated.

5. On the exhale, the stretcher moves his arm farther into extension, then into adduction, and then into internal rotation and pronation. Remember, we want a blend of all three directions to keep moving in a diagonal line. Support the arm but do not push to deepen the stretch.

6. Repeat two to three times.

Sheath Sword Self-Stretch

1. Attach a stretching strap to a fixed object at the floor and behind you. To use a cable and pulley machine at the gym, select the maximum weight so that you cannot lift it. Stand (or sit on a stability ball) so that you can reach your right arm behind and across your back, and rotate so that the little-finger side of your loose fist is against your buttock. Grab on to the stretching strap or the handle of the machine. This is the start of the "sheath sword" position (figure 5.32, p. 106).

2. Start slowly with rotation and then pull forward and out, as if you were reaching for something in front of you. Use the stretching strap to resist this attempt at motion, and hold this isometric contraction for 6 seconds. Then relax and breathe.

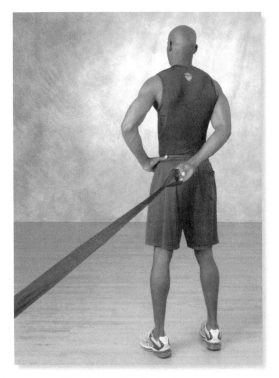

Figure 5.32 "Sheath sword" self-stretch.

3. As you exhale, reach farther behind and across your back, then turn your arm a little more to deepen the stretch on the target muscles. Focus on stretching out of the shoulder joint, and keep your back flat as you stretch. Take up any slack on the stretching strap or reposition yourself at the cable machine, and repeat the sequence two to three times.

Grab Seat Belt Stretch (Flexion End of D1)

This stretch is for increasing range of motion in flexion, adduction, and external rotation.

1. The stretcher is supine, with his right shoulder in as much flexion, adduction, and external rotation as possible, as if reaching for a seat belt. The stretcher keeps his elbow straight and both shoulder blades on the table. His forearm is supinated, and his wrist and fingers are in neutral. To gain as much adduction and flexion as possible, have the stretcher turn his head toward the left shoulder so his chin does not interfere with his arm motion. Ideally, the right upper arm lies across the cheek. This position lengthens the target muscles to their end range. These include the infraspinatus, middle

trapezius, rhomboids, teres minor, posterior deltoid, and pronator teres.

2. Stand at the head of the table to support and stabilize the arm and wrist (figure 5.33). Remember, your hand contacts give the stretcher proprioceptive cues about which way to push or pull. Your hand positions should match your verbal commands. Your grasp spans the wrist and hand and across the elbow to minimize stress on the joints.

3. Direct the stretcher to begin slowly to try to initiate the D1 extension pattern, first with internal rotation, then abduction, then extension. ("Pretend you're pulling your seat belt.")

4. After the isometric push, the stretcher relaxes and inhales deeply. As he relaxes, maintain the arm in the starting position.

5. As he exhales, the stretcher moves the arm farther into flexion, then into adduction, and then into external rotation and supination. Remember, we want a blend of all three directions to keep moving in a diagonal line. Be sure he keeps his shoulder blades on the table so that the stretch comes as he reaches from the shoulder joint. Support the arm but do not push to deepen the stretch.

6. Repeat two to three times.

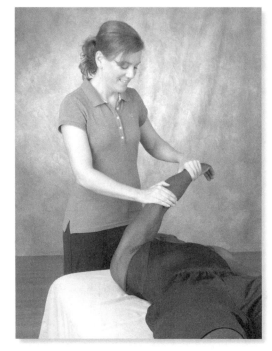

Figure 5.33 Initiation of the "grab seat belt" stretch (D1 pattern). The arm is flexed, adducted, and externally rotated.

Grab Seat Belt Self-Stretch

1. Attach a stretching strap to a fixed object above and behind you. To use a cable and pulley machine at the gym, select the maximum weight so that you cannot lift it. Stand (or sit on a stability ball) so that you can reach your right arm up, across, and rotated as if you were reaching for your seat belt. Grab on to the stretching strap or the handle of the machine. Keep your torso from twisting by focusing on stretching from the shoulder joint. This is the start of the "grab seat belt" stretch (figure 5.34).

2. Start slowly and rotate, then pull down and out, as if you were going to fasten the seat belt. Use the stretching strap to resist this attempt at motion, and hold this isometric contraction for 6 seconds. Then relax and breathe.

3. As you exhale, reach up and across, then rotate your arm a little more to deepen the stretch on the target muscles. Focus on stretching out of the shoulder joint, and keep your torso from twisting. Take up any slack on the stretch-

ing strap or reposition yourself at the cable machine, and repeat the sequence two to three times.

Fasten Seat Belt Stretch (Extension End of D1)

This stretch is used to improve range of motion in extension, abduction, and internal rotation.

1. The stretcher lies supine, with his shoulder joint line at the edge of the table. He has his right shoulder in extension, abduction, and internal rotation as far as possible. His forearm is pronated, with his wrist and fingers in neutral. This position lengthens the target muscles to their end range. These include the pectorals (clavicular head), anterior deltoid, coracobrachialis, biceps brachii, infraspinatus, and supinator.

2. Support and stabilize the arm and wrist (figure 5.35). Your grasp spans the wrist and hand and the elbow to minimize stress on the joints. Remember, your hand contacts give the stretcher proprioceptive cues about which way to push or pull. Your hand positions should match your verbal commands.

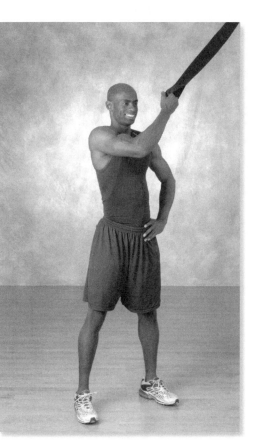

Figure 5.34   "Grab seat belt" self-stretch.

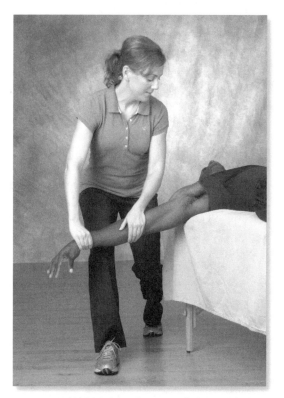

Figure 5.35   **Initiation of the "fasten seat belt" stretch (D1 pattern). The arm is extended, abducted, and internally rotated.**

UPPER EXTREMITY SPIRAL PATTERNS

3. Direct the stretcher to begin slowly to try to initiate the D1 flexion pattern, first with external rotation, then adduction, then flexion. ("Begin by rotating, then push up and across toward your left shoulder.") The stretcher is not attempting to bend his elbow.

4. After the isometric push, the stretcher relaxes and inhales deeply. As he relaxes, maintain the arm in the starting position.

5. As he exhales, the stretcher moves the arm farther into extension, then into abduction, and then internal rotation and pronation. Remember, we want a blend of all three directions to keep moving in a diagonal line. Support the arm but do not push to deepen the stretch.

6. Repeat two to three times.

Fasten Seat Belt Self-Stretch

1. Attach a stretching strap to a fixed object at the floor and behind you. To use a cable and pulley machine at the gym, select the maximum weight so that you cannot lift it. Stand (or sit on a stability ball) so that you can reach your right arm behind and away from you, and rotate so that your thumb faces behind you as if you were putting on a seat belt. Grab on to the stretching strap or the handle of the machine. This is the start of the "fasten seat belt" position (figure 5.36).

2. Start slowly with rotation, then pull forward and in as if you were reaching up and across to your opposite shoulder to grab a seat belt. Use the stretching strap to resist this attempt at motion, and hold this isometric contraction for 6 seconds. Then relax and breathe.

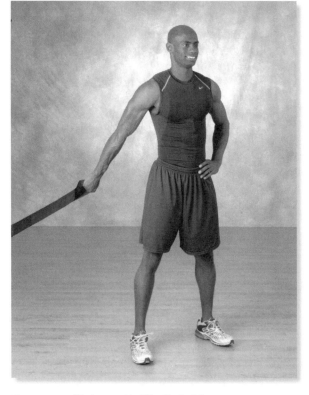

Figure 5.36 "Fasten seat belt" self-stretch.

3. As you exhale, reach farther behind and away from you, then turn your arm a little more to deepen the stretch on the target muscles. Focus on stretching out of the shoulder joint, and keep your back flat as you stretch. Take up any slack on the stretching strap or reposition yourself at the cable machine, and repeat the sequence two to three times.

Stretches for the Neck and Torso

This chapter addresses the muscles of the torso and neck. Most people carry excess tension in the neck and low back area, so facilitated stretching techniques are a quick and simple way to provide more ease and comfort in these core areas.

The nature of our daily lives requires a great deal of flexion in the torso and neck—we sit at desks, in cars, in front of the computer and television. Our chairs are not really designed to support our bodies well, and the postural muscles are called upon to literally "take up the slack." Most sports also require a great deal of support and active involvement from these muscles. The following stretches can be used as preventive techniques or to help relieve pain caused by imbalance in these muscles.

Muscles of the Neck

Anatomy

The cervical, or neck, area is a storehouse of muscular tension. Many people experience discomfort or pain in this region because of postural stress, job-related activities, or trauma. Stretching the neck muscles can provide great relief from tightness and pain but can also create pain if done too aggressively.

When performing these stretches, be especially careful that the stretcher is pain free at all times. If you are working with someone who has suffered any type of neck injury, work cautiously. Sometimes the stretcher may not realize that he is overworking and will end up with increased pain a day or two later.

Muscles of the cervical region include the upper trapezius, sternocleidomastoid (SCM), suboccipitals, scalenes, and levator scapulae. We discuss each here, then describe the functional assessment of the cervical spine.

▪ *Upper trapezius*—Many people have upper trapezius muscles that are hypertonic. When the upper trapezius muscles are too tight, they can cause headaches and pain. They also develop significant trigger points.

▪ *Sternocleidomastoid*—The SCM is a complex muscle with many actions. At its inferior attachments, it has two parts, the sternal and clavicular. These two divisions merge into a common attachment on the skull.

▪ *Suboccipitals*—The four suboccipital muscles comprise two pairs: the two rectus capitis and the two obliquus muscles. They are the deepest muscles of the posterior upper neck. The rectus capitis posterior major and the obliques form the "suboccipital triangle" on each side of the spine. The vertebral artery crosses through the triangle, which is filled with dense, fatty connective tissue and is covered by the more superficial semispinalis capitis and longissimus capitis. Even though they are small, these muscles often hold a tremendous amount of tension and benefit greatly from stretching.

▪ *Scalenes*—The scalene muscles are divided into three sections: anterior, middle, and posterior. They are strongly implicated in thoracic outlet syndrome, carpal tunnel syndrome,

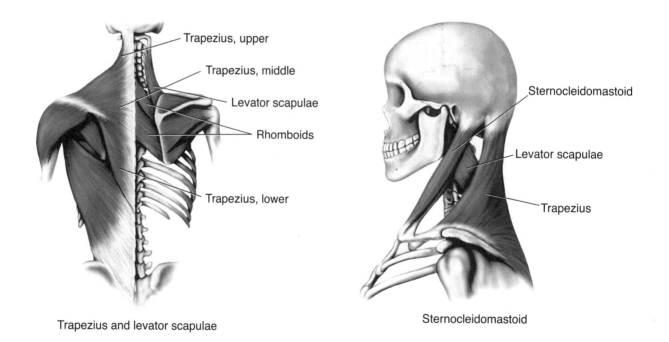

Trapezius, upper

Trapezius, middle

Levator scapulae

Rhomboids

Trapezius, lower

Trapezius and levator scapulae

Sternocleidomastoid

Levator scapulae

Trapezius

Sternocleidomastoid

and other painful conditions of the neck, shoulder, and arm. This is so because the brachial plexus (a bundle of nerves) and the subclavian artery pass between the anterior and middle scalenes and may become entrapped and compromised if the muscles are hypertonic.

▌ *Levator scapulae*—The levator scapulae is often implicated in complaints of neck stiffness, especially when rotation is limited. Postural stress may cause this muscle to be hypertonic or eccentrically stressed, in which case it may need strengthening rather than stretching.

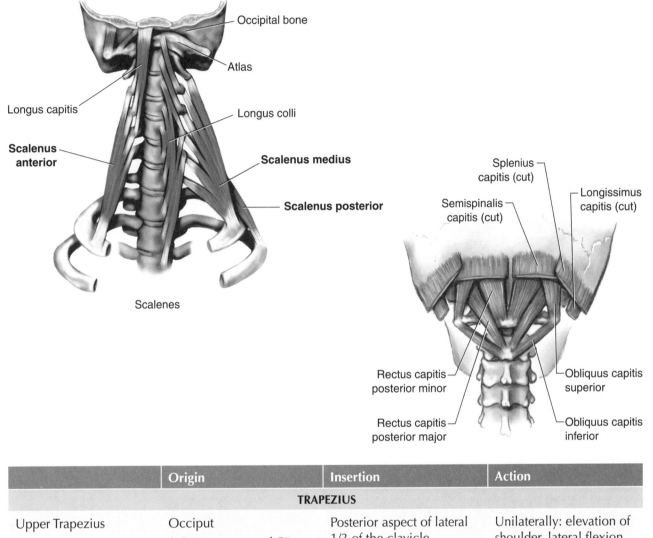

MUSCLES OF THE NECK

	Origin	Insertion	Action
TRAPEZIUS			
Upper Trapezius	Occiput Spinous process of C7-T12 and the ligamentum nuchae	Posterior aspect of lateral 1/3 of the clavicle	Unilaterally: elevation of shoulder, lateral flexion of head and neck Bilaterally: extension of head and neck
STERNOCLEIDOMASTOID			
Sternocleidomastoid	Sternal division: anterior aspect of manubrium of sternum Clavicular division: anterior, superior aspect of medial 1/3 of the clavicle	Lateral aspect of mastoid process Lateral half of superior nuchal line on the occipital bone	Bilaterally: flexion of head and neck, especially against resistance of gravity Unilaterally: rotation of head to opposite side, assists lateral flexion to same side

(continued)

MUSCLES OF THE NECK

	Origin	Insertion	Action
SCALENES			
Anterior scalene	Anterior aspect of transverse processes of C3-C6	Superior aspect of 1st rib	Lateral flexion of cervical spine Assists neck flexion Elevates ribs during inspiration
Middle scalene	Transverse processes of C2-C7	Superior aspect of the 1st rib posterior to middle scalene	Lateral flexion of cerivcal spine Elevates ribs during inspiration
Posterior scalene	Transverse processes of C5-C7	Superior aspect of the 2nd rib posterior to middle scalene	Lateral flexion of cervical spine Elevates ribs during inspiration
LEVATOR SCAPULAE			
Levator Scapulae	Transverse process of C1-C4	Superior angle and medial border of scapula	Bilaterally: extends head and neck, assists shoulder shrugs Unilaterally: assists downward rotation and elevation of scapula, assists lateral flexion and rotation of neck to same side
SUBOCCIPITALS			
Rectus capitis posterior (RCP) major	Spinous process of the axis (C2)	Inferior nuchal line of the occiput, lateral to the RCP minor	Extends the head on the neck Rotates and tilts the head to the same side
Rectus capitis posterior (RCP) minor	Tubercle located on the posterior arch of the atlas (C1)	Inferior nuchal line of the occiput, medial to the RCP major	Extends the head on the neck
Obliquus capitis superior	Transverse process of the atlas (C1)	Lateral aspect of the occiput, between the superior and inferior nuchal lines	Extends the head on the neck Tilts the head to the same side
Obliquus capitis inferior	Spinous process of the axis (C2)	Transverse process of the axis (C1)	Rotates and tilts the head to the same side

Functional Assessment

The cervical spine is capable of motion in six directions: flexion, extension, lateral flexion to each side, and rotation to each side. These motions can also be combined to create a greater variety of movement. In addition to moving with the neck, the head moves independently on the cervical spine in flexion, extension, rotation, and tilting to the side (figure 6.1).

Movement of the head and neck is more complex than movements around other joints. Many muscles contribute to each movement, and it is difficult to isolate one muscle at a time. Therefore, even though our focus is on five groups (upper trapezius, SCM,

ROM for the Head on the Neck

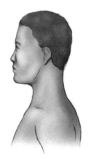
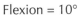
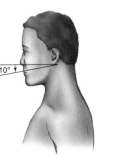
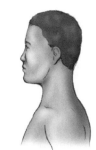
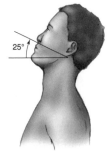

Flexion = 10°   Extension = 25°

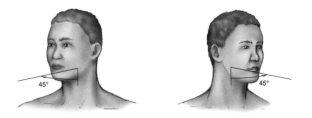

Rotation = 45°

ROM for the Neck

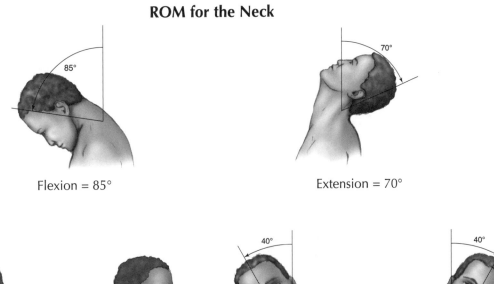

Flexion = 85°   Extension = 70°

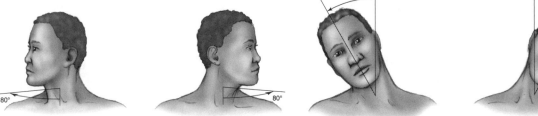

Rotation = 80°   Lateral flexion = 40°

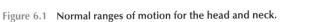

Figure 6.1   Normal ranges of motion for the head and neck.

suboccipitals, scalenes, and levator scapulae), synergistic muscles that contribute to the same motion will also be affected.

Range of motion for the head on the neck is as follows:

Flexion = 10 degrees (tucking chin to neck)
Extension = 25 degrees (looking up)
Rotation = 45 degrees

Range of motion for the neck is as follows (these values include the motion of the head on the neck in the previous list):

Flexion = 85 degrees
Extension = 70 degrees
Rotation = 80 degrees
Lateral flexion = 40 degrees

 ### Upper Trapezius Stretch, Supine, With a Partner

This stretch is used to improve range of motion in cervical rotation and flexion and shoulder depression.

1. The stretcher is supine. Help her rotate her head to the right as far as possible without pain, then tuck her chin as far as possible. If the right shoulder interferes with this motion, have the stretcher pull it down, away from the head, and tuck the chin again. The stretcher also pulls her left shoulder down away from her head. This starting position lengthens the left upper trapezius to its pain-free end range.

2. Place your left hand at the stretcher's occiput, fingers pointing toward the ceiling. Place your right hand on her left shoulder (figure 6.2). Ask

the stretcher to begin slowly to push against both of your hands, as if bringing the back of her head and her left shoulder together. You provide matching resistance as she isometrically contracts her left upper trapezius for 6 seconds. She is pushing equally from both ends and breathing normally throughout.

3. After the isometric push, the stretcher relaxes and breathes in. As she relaxes, maintain the head in the starting position.

4. As she exhales, the stretcher rotates her head farther to the right, tucks her chin more (if possible), and pulls her left shoulder farther away from her head. This deepens the upper trapezius stretch.

5. Repeat two to three times.

Upper Trapezius Stretch, With a Partner, Supine Arm Pull

This is an alternate stretch, easier to perform, but slightly less effective than the previous protocol.

1. The stretcher is supine on the table. Stand at her left side and ask her to reach her left arm toward her feet to depress the left shoulder. Grasp the left hand and wrist. This starting position lengthens the left upper trapezius (figure 6.3).

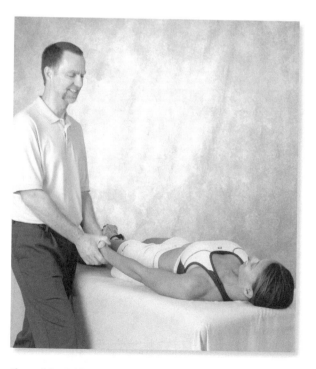
Figure 6.3 Initiation of the left upper trapezius stretch, using the arm.

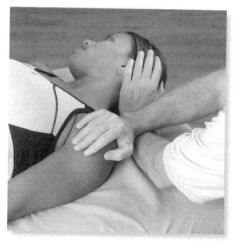
Figure 6.2 Initiation of the left upper trapezius stretch.

2. Direct the stretcher to slowly attempt to shrug her left shoulder while you prevent the motion. Hold this isometric contraction of the upper trapezius for 6 seconds.

3. The stretcher relaxes and breathes, and as she exhales, ask her to reach toward her feet again, deepening the stretch on her left upper trapezius.

4. Repeat two to three times.

Upper Trapezius Self-Stretch, Supine

1. This is an easy stretch to do by yourself. Lie down on your back, keep your neck lengthened, and turn your head to the right as far as possible; tuck your chin as far as possible, and pull your left shoulder toward your feet. Now, place your left arm under your body to anchor your left shoulder. Wrap your right arm around your head so that your right fingers can hold the base of your skull (figure 6.4).

2. From this starting position, try to bring your left shoulder and the back of your head toward each other for 6 seconds while you resist the motion with your hands.

3. Following this isometric contraction of the left upper trapezius, increase the stretch by turning farther to the right, tucking your chin, and pulling your left shoulder farther away from your head.

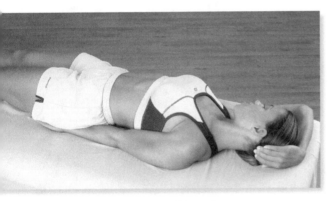

Figure 6.4 **Upper trapezius self-stretch.**

Sternocleidomastoid Stretch, Supine, With a Partner

This stretch is used to improve rotation of the head and neck.

1. The stretcher is supine. Keeping her neck lengthened, guide her as she rotates her head to the left as far as possible without pain. This

starting position lengthens the left SCM to its pain-free end range.

2. Cradle the stretcher's head in your left hand, which rests on the table; place your right hand just above her right ear (figure 6.5). Ask the client to begin slowly to attempt to rotate her head to the right. She is not trying to lift her head from the table. You provide matching resistance as she isometrically contracts her SCM for 6 seconds. The client is breathing normally throughout.

3. After the isometric push, the stretcher relaxes and breathes in. As she relaxes, maintain the head in the starting position.

4. As she exhales, the stretcher rotates her head farther to the left, deepening the stretch on the left SCM.

5. Repeat two to three times.

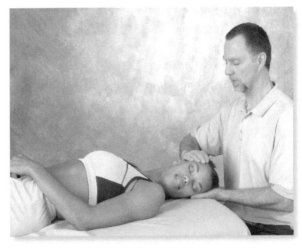

Figure 6.5 **Initiation of the sternocleidomastoid stretch.**

Sternocleidomastoid Self-Stretch, Supine

1. Lie down on your back and turn your head to the left as far as possible, keeping your neck lengthened. Place one hand under your head and the other just above your right ear.

2. From this starting position, begin slowly, and attempt to turn your head to the right for 6 seconds while you resist the motion with your hands. Be sure not to try to lift your head from the floor or table; only turn to the right (figure 6.6, p. 116).

3. After this isometric contraction of the SCM, relax, breathe, and increase the stretch by turning farther to the left.

MUSCLES OF THE NECK

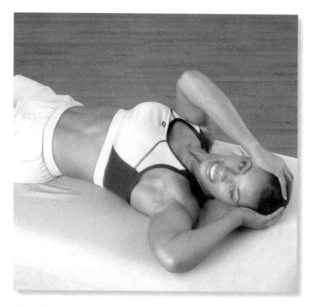

Figure 6.6 **Sternocleidomastoid self-stretch. Keep your head on the table.**

🔵 Scalenes Stretch, Supine, With a Partner

This stretch is for improving lateral flexion of the head and neck.

1. The stretcher is supine. Guide her as she laterally flexes her head and neck to the right as far as possible without pain. Prevent her from adding rotation to the motion by asking her to keep her nose pointed directly at the ceiling. She also pulls her left shoulder away from her head to anchor the attachments of the scalenes on the ribs. This starting position lengthens the left scalenes to their pain-free end range.

✋ 2. Place your right hand on the stretcher's head just above her left ear. Place your left hand against her left shoulder to anchor it in place (figure 6.7). Direct the stretcher to begin slowly to push against your right hand as if she is trying to bring her left ear directly to her left shoulder. Be sure she does not add rotation to her effort. She does not push up with her shoulder because we're using the shoulder to anchor the ribs, which are the distal attachment of the scalenes. You provide matching resistance as she isometrically contracts her scalenes for 6 seconds. The stretcher is breathing normally throughout.

3. After the isometric push, the stretcher relaxes and breathes in. As she relaxes, maintain the head in the starting position.

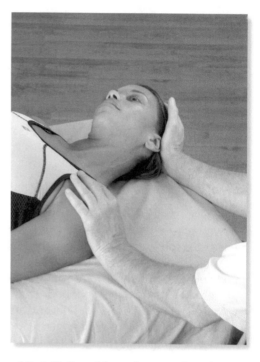

Figure 6.7 **Initiation of the scalene stretch, with no rotation of the head.**

🔄 4. As she exhales, ask the stretcher to bring her right ear closer to her right shoulder, being sure to keep her nose pointed directly at the ceiling. This deepens the stretch of the left scalenes.

⚠️ 5. Repeat two to three times, then help the stretcher reposition her head to do the same stretch for the right scalenes.

For more specificity, you can isolate the anterior or posterior scalenes by rotating the head as follows:

▪ *Left anterior scalene*—Laterally flex the neck to the right, then rotate the head 45 degrees to the left. From this position, follow the stretching sequence (figure 6.8*a*).

▪ *Left posterior scalene*—Laterally flex the neck to the right, then rotate the head 45 degrees to the right. From this position, follow the stretching sequence (figure 6.8*b*).

▪ *Right anterior scalene*—Laterally flex the neck to the left, then rotate the head 45 degrees to the right. From this position, follow the stretching sequence (figure 6.8*c*).

▪ *Right posterior scalene*—Laterally flex the neck to the left, then rotate the head 45 degrees to the left. From this position, follow the stretching sequence (figure 6.8*d*).

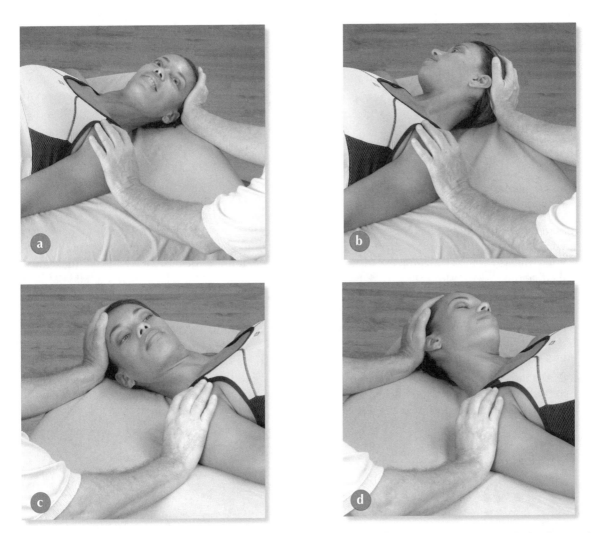

Figure 6.8 **Isolating the scalenes.** *(a)* **Left anterior scalene,** *(b)* **left posterior scalene,** *(c)* **right anterior scalene, and** *(d)* **right posterior scalene.**

Scalenes Self-Stretch, Supine

1. Lie down on your back. Pull your left shoulder away from your ear and anchor it by placing your left arm under your body. Keeping your nose pointed toward the ceiling (so you don't rotate your head), side-bend your neck to bring your right ear as close to your right shoulder as possible. You may need to lift your head slightly as you move, if it won't slide on the floor. Once you've completed the side-bend, let your head rest on the floor again. Bring your right arm up around your head, with your fingers holding just above your left ear (figure 6.9).

2. From this starting position, try to bring your left ear toward your left shoulder. Don't try to lift your head from the floor as you push, and keep your nose pointed at the ceiling. After this 6-second isometric contraction of the left

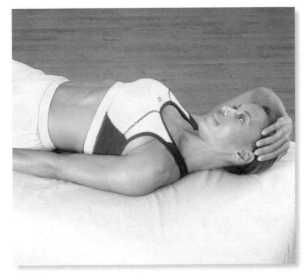

Figure 6.9 **Scalenes self-stretch. Keep your head on the table as you push.**

scalenes, see if you can bring your right ear closer to your right shoulder. Don't pull it with your hand; use your neck muscles. You may need to lift your head slightly as you move, if it won't slide on the floor.

Suboccipitals Stretch, Supine, With a Partner

This stretch is used to help improve flexion of the head on the neck and to release the head to balance more freely on the cervical spine.

1. The stretcher is supine. Sit at her head and cup your hands under the head so that the pads of your fingers (not the fingertips) can palpate the occiput. Ask the stretcher to tuck her chin toward her throat. She does not try to lift her head toward her chest; rather, she is trying to lengthen the back of her neck. This starting position lengthens the suboccipitals to their end range (figure 6.10, a & b).

2. Direct the stretcher to begin slowly and gently to tilt her head back. As she begins, you may feel the occiput slip from your fingers. If this happens, stop and start again, very slowly, so that you can maintain contact with the occiput. This isometric contraction can be done with a minimum of effort by the stretcher. Hold for 6 seconds as the stretcher breathes normally.

3. The stretcher relaxes and breathes, and as she exhales, tucks her chin again, deepening the stretch on the suboccipitals.

4. Repeat one to two times.

Suboccipitals Self-Stretch, Supine

1. Lie on your back and wrap your hands around the back of your head so that your thumbs are sitting at the base of your skull. Tuck your chin into your throat, trying not to lift your head off the floor (figure 6.11).

2. From this starting position, gently try to tilt your head back, using your thumbs to prevent the motion. Hold this isometric contraction of the suboccipitals for 6 seconds. Relax and breathe, and as you exhale, tuck your chin again, deepening the stretch on the suboccipitals.

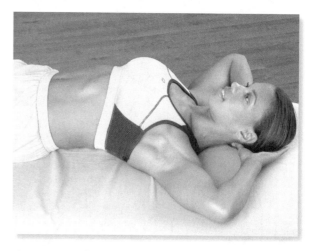

Figure 6.11 **Suboccipitals self-stretch.**

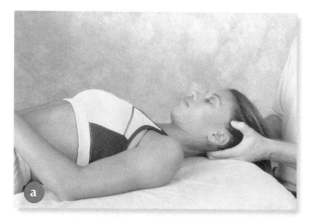

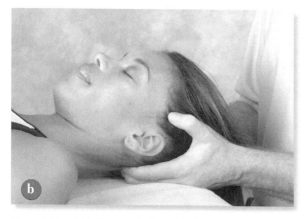

Figure 6.10 *(a)* **Initiation of suboccipitals stretch and** *(b)* **illustration of finger placement.**

Levator Scapulae Stretch, With a Partner, Sitting

This stretch is used to improve head and neck flexion and to help normalize the position of the shoulder blade on the back.

1. The stretcher sits comfortably on a chair or low stool, keeping her back lengthened. Ask her to tuck her chin to her chest and then rotate her head to the right about 45 degrees. Stand behind the stretcher, and place one hand on

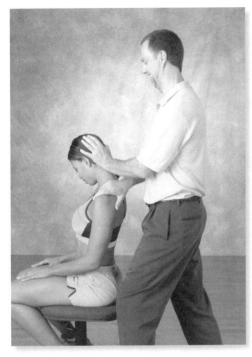

Figure 6.12   **Initiation of levator scapulae stretch.**

Levator Scapulae Self-Stretch, Sitting

1. Sit comfortably, keeping your spine lengthened. Use your muscles to pull your left shoulder blade down your back and hold it there. Drop your head to your chest, then turn your chin to the right about 45 degrees. Bring your right hand up to the top of your head and pull slightly until you feel a stretch of the left levator scapulae. You may need to play with your head position a little to find this place of stretch. Be sure to keep your spine long (figure 6.13).

2. From this starting position, slowly try to lift your head and neck against your own resistance, isometrically contracting the left levator scapulae for 6 seconds. Relax and breathe, and as you exhale, increase the stretch by tucking your chin more.

3. Repeat two to three times.

the back of her head and the other at the top of her left scapula. This starting position lengthens the left levator to its end range (figure 6.12).

2. Direct the stretcher to start slowly to try to lift her head and neck and her left shoulder simultaneously as you provide resistance to this isometric contraction of the left levator for 6 seconds. Be sure the stretcher is not just trying to extend the head on the neck, but is lifting the head and neck together.

3. At the end of the isometric push, the stretcher relaxes and breathes, and as she exhales, tucks her chin closer to her chest to deepen the stretch on the levator.

4. Repeat two to three times.

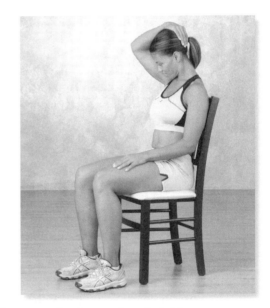

Figure 6.13   **Levator scapulae self-stretch.**

MUSCLES OF THE NECK

Muscles of the Torso

Anatomy

The thoracic and lumbar areas often maintain chronic muscular tension, which can be greatly alleviated through effective stretching. Many people experience pain in these areas from trauma, job-related injury, or postural stress. When performing these stretches, be especially aware that the stretcher is working in the pain-free zone at all times. If you are working with someone who has suffered any type of back injury, work cautiously. Sometimes the stretcher may not realize he is overworking and will have increased pain a day or two after stretching.

The back extensors, trunk rotators, quadratus lumborum, and latissimus dorsi support the thoracic and lumbar spine.

▌ *Back extensors*—The back extensors consist of the erector spinae group (iliocostalis, longissimus, and spinalis, each with two or three divisions) and the transversospinalis group (semispinalis thoracis, multifidus, rotatores, interspinales, and intertransversarii). We illustrate the erector spinae here but are not listing the origins and insertions. These muscles, acting bilaterally, extend the spine. Acting unilaterally, they assist trunk rotation. When they are hypertonic, they can create back pain and limit spinal flexion and rotation. They are also common sites for trigger points.

▌ *Trunk rotators*—Trunk rotation involves the thoracic and lumbar spine. The major muscles of rotation are the internal and external oblique abdominal muscles, assisted by the erector spinae, semispinalis thoracis, multifidus, and rotatores. We are listing only the oblique abdominal muscles here. The external oblique angles downward and medially from the ribs. The internal oblique angles upward and medially from the lateral and posterior iliac crest.

▌ *Quadratus lumborum*—The quadratus lumborum (QL) is an important component of a strong and

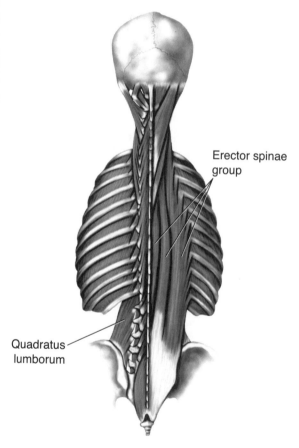

Erector spinae group

Quadratus lumborum

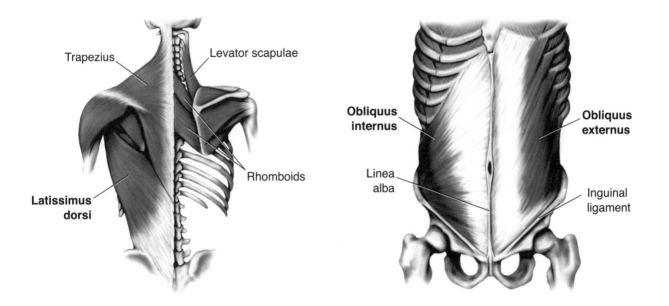

Trapezius

Levator scapulae

Rhomboids

Latissimus dorsi

Obliquus internus

Obliquus externus

Linea alba

Inguinal ligament

healthy low back. When this muscle is hypertonic, it develops trigger points that refer pain to the hips, to the gluteal area, and down the leg. The QL is always involved in low back pain, even that resulting from disc problems or misalignment of the lumbar vertebrae.

▮ *Latissimus dorsi*—Latissimus dorsi forms part of the posterior axillary border and is used in many activities in which the arm moves from overhead downward, like chopping wood, swimming, and rock climbing. It's often overlooked as a source of back pain.

Muscle	Origin	Insertion	Action
OBLIQUE ABDOMINAL MUSCLES (TRUNK ROTATORS)			
External oblique	Lateral and inferior aspects of the lower eight ribs	Anterior iliac crest and linea alba via the abdominal aponeurosis	Bilaterally: increase intra-abdominal pressure, trunk flexion Unilaterally: lateral flexion of trunk to same side, rotation of trunk to opposite side
Internal oblique	Thoracolumbar fascia Anterior and lateral iliac crest Lateral half of inguinal ligament	Cartilage of the lower three ribs Linea alba via the abdominal aponeurosis	Bilaterally: increase intra-abdominal pressure, trunk flexion Unilaterally: lateral flexion and rotation of trunk to same side

(continued)

MUSCLES OF THE TORSO

Muscle	Origin	Insertion	Action
QUADRATUS LUMBORUM			
Quadratus lumborum	Posterior iliac crest and iliolumbar ligament	Inferior border of the 12th rib and transverse processes of L1-L5	Bilaterally: stabilizes the 12th rib during respiration, assists extension of lumbar spine Unilaterally: lateral flexion of trunk or elevation of ilium
LATISSIMUS DORSI			
Latissimus dorsi	Spinous processes of T7-L5 Sacrum via the lumbar aponeurosis Crest of ilium	Medial aspect of bicipital groove of humerus	Extension of arm from a flexed position Adduction Shoulder depression Assists internal rotation Provides a "vest pocket" for inferior angle of scapula, holding it against ribs

Functional Assessment

Trunk motion is a combination of movement at the lumbar and thoracic spine (figure 6.14). Six directions are possible: flexion, extension, rotation to each side, and lateral flexion to each side. These movements can also be combined to create a greater variety of motion.

Movement in the lumbar and thoracic spine is a complex combination of motion at each vertebra. Many muscles contribute to every motion, and it is difficult to isolate one muscle at a time. Therefore, even though our focus is on the major muscles of the trunk region, smaller muscles that contribute to the same motion will also be affected.

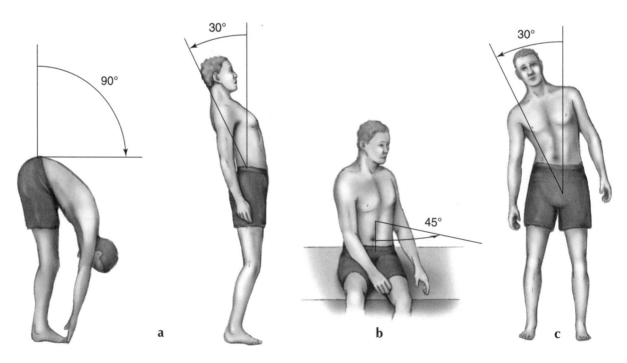

Figure 6.14 **Normal thoracolumbar ranges of motion.** *(a)* Flexion-extension, *(b)* rotation, and *(c)* lateral flexion.

The thoracolumbar range of motion is as follows:

Flexion = 90 degrees

Extension = 30 degrees

Rotation = 45 degrees

Lateral flexion = 30 degrees

Trunk Rotators (Oblique Abdominal Muscles) Stretch, With a Partner, Sitting

Twisting to the right stretches the right external oblique and the left internal oblique.

1. The stretcher is seated on the table, with his knees bent and legs hanging over the side. This position stabilizes the hips. Keeping his spine lengthened and without arching his back, he twists to the right as far as he can, keeping his nose in alignment with his sternum (this neutral position is more comfortable). This position lengthens the left trunk rotators to their pain-free end range.

2. Reach under the stretcher's right arm to place your right hand on his anterior shoulder. Place your left hand on his left scapula, near the inferomedial border. Ask him to begin slowly to twist back to the left, keeping his head in neutral (figure 6.15). Be sure he is twisting from his trunk and not just pushing back with his shoulder. You provide matching resistance for this isometric contraction, being sure that the client is breathing normally throughout.

3. After the isometric push, the stretcher relaxes and breathes in. As he relaxes, he maintains his torso in the starting position.

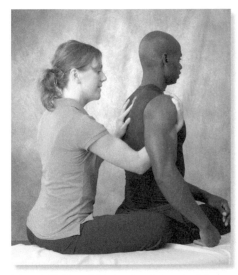

Figure 6.15 **Initiation of the trunk rotators stretch.**

4. As he exhales, ask him to rotate farther to the right, keeping his head in neutral and his spine lengthened. This increases the stretch of the left trunk rotators.

5. Repeat two to three times, then reposition the client to do the same stretch for the right trunk rotators.

Trunk Rotators (Oblique Abdominal Muscles) Self-Stretch, Sitting

1. Sit comfortably in a straight-back chair. Keeping your spine lengthened and your head in neutral, twist to the left as far as you can, then grab the back of the chair to hold yourself there.

2. From this starting position, try to twist back to the right, using your trunk, not just your shoulders. Hold this isometric contraction of the obliques for 6 seconds, and keep breathing normally.

3. After this isometric contraction, take a deep breath, and as you exhale, twist farther to the left, using your trunk and not pulling with your arms, to stretch the obliques (figure 6.16).

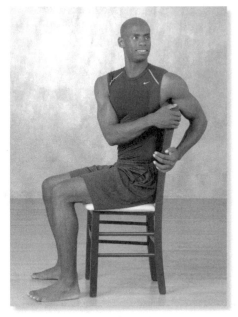

Figure 6.16 **Trunk rotators self-stretch.**

Quadratus Lumborum Stretch, Side-Lying, With a Partner

The QL is a muscle with many functions. It laterally flexes (side-bends) the trunk and elevates the hip. It also helps to stabilize the low back and is therefore usually involved when low back pain is present. The QL has fibers that run vertically and in two diagonals.

This stretch is primarily for the vertical fibers, which make up the bulk of the muscle. It works best if the hip abductors are stretched first (see pp. 47-50).

1. The stretcher is lying on his left side, with his back at the edge of the table and his right leg hyperextended and hanging over the edge of the table. He has his left leg bent and as close to his chest as possible. Be sure he keeps his hips stacked vertically on top of each other. He reaches his right arm up over his head. This lengthens the right QL. If the stretcher experiences any low back pain in this position, he may bend forward from the waist to round his low back while keeping his leg hanging off the edge of the table.

2. Stand behind the stretcher. Cross your arms and place your left hand against his right iliac crest; your right hand is spread wide and placed on the lateral aspect of his rib cage (figure 6.17). This crossed-hands position gives you a better mechanical advantage to resist the isometric contraction of QL.

3. Stretcher education begins now. Your goal is to have the stretcher contract the right QL by bringing the hip and the ribs toward each other. He is side-bending and "hiking" his hip at the same time. Many people have difficulty doing this, so you may need to break the motion into separate components and work with him until he can do each motion separately, then combine them. Be patient and creative.

4. Once the stretcher can perform the motion, ask him to begin slowly to try to bring the top of his hip and his rib cage toward each other.

You apply matching resistance to prevent any motion from occurring. You control the force of his effort.

5. After the isometric push, the stretcher relaxes and inhales deeply. As he relaxes, allow his leg (and his hip) to drop toward the floor.

6. As he exhales, ask the client to pull his foot closer to the floor and reach farther up over his head to increase the stretch on the right QL.

7. Repeat two to three times.

Quadratus Lumborum Stretch, Supine, With a Partner, Leg Pull

This version of the QL stretch, though slightly less effective, is easier for both the stretcher and the partner.

1. The stretcher is supine on the table. The partner firmly grasps the right foot and ankle and passively stretches the entire leg to pull the hip down, then across the midline, lengthening the QL on the right (figure 6.18).

2. From this starting position, the stretcher attempts to "hip hike" (pull the hipbone toward the head). Be sure he is not lifting the leg toward the ceiling (hip flexion). Hold this isometric contraction of the QL for 6 seconds as the stretcher breathes normally.

3. After the isometric push, the stretcher relaxes and inhales deeply. As he relaxes, maintain the leg in the starting position.

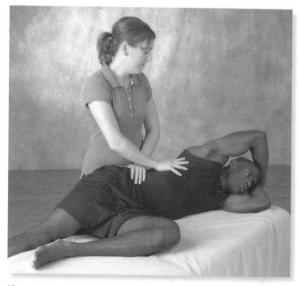

Figure 6.17 Initiation of the quadratus lumborum stretch.

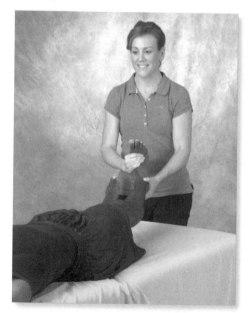

Figure 6.18 Initiation of the quadratus lumborum stretch, using the leg.

4. As he exhales, passively stretch the leg down and across the midline farther, deepening the stretch on the right QL.

 5. Repeat two to three times.

 ## Quadratus Lumborum Self-Stretch, Sitting Side-Bend

1. Sit comfortably, with your spine lengthened. Place a towel or stretching strap under your left foot, and hold the other end in your left hand. Side-bend to the left as far as you can, taking up any slack in the stretching strap. This lengthens the right QL (figure 6.19).

2. Using the stretching strap to prevent your motion, try to sit up straight, isometrically contracting the right QL for 6 seconds as you keep breathing normally.

3. After the isometric contraction, relax, breathe, and deepen the stretch by bending farther to the left.

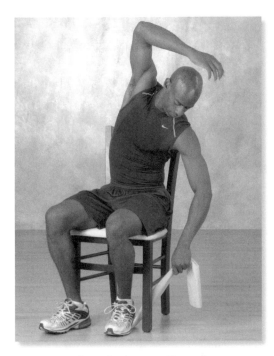

Figure 6.19 **Quadratus lumborum self-stretch.**

 ## Latissimus Dorsi Stretch, Prone, With a Partner

This stretch, which mimics the "lat pull-down" used to strengthen the latissimus dorsi, increases range of motion in flexion and external rotation of the humerus.

1. The stretcher is prone on the table, with his arms outstretched (in the "superman" position) and externally rotated (thumbs up). This position lengthens the latissimus dorsi to their end range.

2. Using a stable front-to-back lunge stance, grasp the stretcher's arms or wrists securely (figure 6.20). Direct the stretcher to begin slowly to try to pull his elbows toward his sides and rotate his arms internally, isometrically contracting the latissimus dorsi bilaterally for 6 seconds.

3. After the isometric pull, the stretcher relaxes and breathes in.

4. As he exhales, ask the stretcher to reach farther forward (away from his feet), toward the ceiling, and externally rotate his arms more, deepening the stretch of the latissimus dorsi.

5. Repeat two to three times.

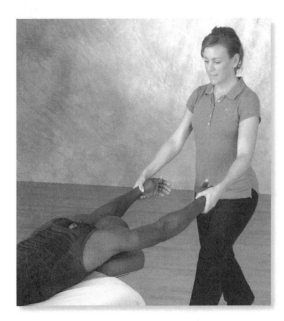

Figure 6.20 **Initiation of the latissimus dorsi stretch.**

 ## Latissimus Dorsi Self-Stretch, Standing, Pull-Up Bar

This stretch utilizes your own body weight to provide resistance during the isometric phase.

1. With your hands at least shoulder-width apart on a pull-up bar, bend your knees and drop toward the floor until your arms are completely stretched out above you and are holding your weight (figure 6.21, p. 126). This position stretches the latissimus dorsi.

MUSCLES OF THE TORSO

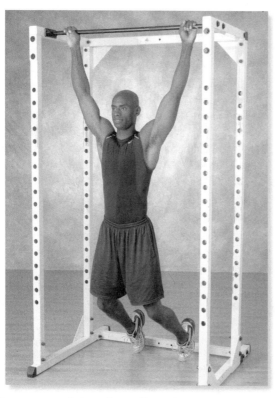

Figure 6.21 Latissimus dorsi self-stretch, standing.

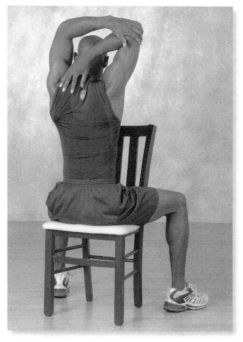

Figure 6.22 Latissimus dorsi self-stretch, sitting.

2. Slowly attempt a pull-up from this position. The goal is simply to engage the latissimus dorsi isometrically, not to complete the pull-up. Hold this isometric contraction for 6 seconds, breathing normally.

3. Relax and breathe. As you exhale, let your body weight drop toward the floor, deepening the stretch on the latissimus dorsi. Repeat two to three times.

Latissimus Dorsi Self-Stretch, Seated

1. This stretch may be done seated or standing, but the seated position stabilizes your hips to help your biomechanics. Keep your back and neck lengthened and bring your right arm, elbow bent, up behind your head, trying to reach your left shoulder. Grab your right elbow with your left hand (figure 6.22).

2. From this starting position, attempt to bring your right arm down to your right side, resisting with your left hand. Hold this isometric contraction of the right latissimus dorsi for 6 seconds, breathing normally.

3. Relax and breathe. Following the isometric contraction, reach your right arm farther to the

left to increase the stretch on the right latissimus dorsi. Repeat two to three times.

4. To increase the stretch even more, side-bend to the left.

Back Extensors Stretch, With a Partner, Sitting

This stretch is used to improve trunk flexion.

1. The stretcher is seated at the edge of the treatment table (or on the floor), with his knees slightly bent (to relax the hamstrings) during this stretch. He leans forward as far as possible by contracting the rectus abdominis and psoas. The stretcher focuses on bending from the hips and not "stooping" in his upper back. He keeps his head in line with his spine or may drop his chin to his chest. This lengthens his back extensors to their pain-free end of range.

2. Place both hands on the stretcher's lower back to provide resistance to the isometric contraction of the back extensors (figure 6.23a).

3. Direct the stretcher to begin slowly to attempt to extend his spine, isometrically contracting the back extensors. He focuses on the part of his spine where your hands are. He does not use his arms to push back. A guide to help with the attempted motion is for him to think of bending backward around your hands.

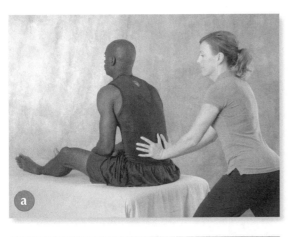

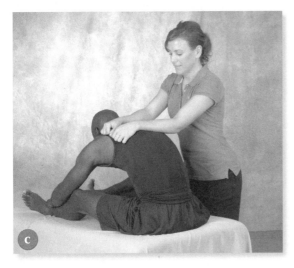

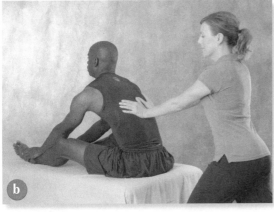

Figure 6.23 *(a)* **Initiation of the back extensors stretch;** *(b)* **applying resistance at the midback; and** *(c)* **applying resistance at the upper back.**

4. After the isometric push, the stretcher relaxes and inhales deeply. During this time, maintain the spine in the starting position.

5. As he exhales, the stretcher contracts his rectus abdominis and psoas to bend farther forward, deepening the stretch of the back extensors.

Remind the stretcher to keep his back lengthened and bend from the hips.

6. Repeat three to five times, each time moving your hands farther up the back. As your hands move up his back, he moves the focus of his isometric contraction to match. Once the focus of the isometric contraction has moved to the midback and upper back, the stretcher may "stoop" and pull his chin to his chest during the stretching phase to fully lengthen the extensors of the midback and upper back area (figure 6.23, *b* & *c*).

Back Extensors Self-Stretch, Seated

1. Sit in a chair and, keeping your upper back straight and bending from the hips, bend forward as far as you can (figure 6.24). Place a folded towel across your lower back and hold on to the ends with each hand.

2. Start slowly and try to bend backward around the towel, isometrically contracting the low back portion of the extensors for 6 seconds.

3. Relax, breathe, and stretch by bending farther forward if you can.

4. Move the towel about 6 inches (15 centimeters) up your back and repeat the sequence. Continue moving the towel in 6-inch increments all the way up the back. As you work your way up to the midback and upper back, you may bend your upper back and pull your chin to your chest to increase the stretch of the midback and upper back extensors.

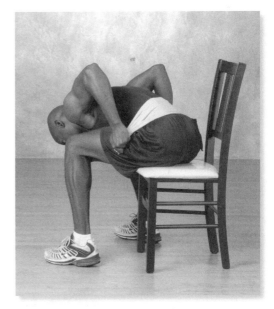

Figure 6.24 **Back extensors self-stretch.**

PART III

Beyond
the Basics

This section of the book contains what we think of as more advanced material. Chapter 7 discusses the use of facilitated stretching in conjunction with massage or other manual therapy techniques and provides examples of possible treatment protocols in six different scenarios.

In chapter 8, we provide suggested stretching routines for five popular athletic activities and two routines for daily use outside of athletics.

In chapter 9, we provide an overview of nine common soft tissue injuries that respond well to a self-directed strengthening and stretching program.

Combining Techniques to Release Fibrotic Tissue

Injured muscles usually heal by forming scar tissue at the injury site. The final scar is often dense and inflexible, limiting pain-free motion. To restore pain-free motion, the scar tissue must be modified in some way. Physicians are generally limited to medication or surgery in their approach to treatment and can do very little about scarring. Many physical therapists still rely on treatments such as ice, heat, ultrasound, and electrical muscle stimulation. These approaches are often effective and many times an important component in the early treatment of soft tissue trauma, but they are inadequate for modifying fully formed scar tissue. Some type of manual therapy, like massage or myofascial release, is necessary to effectively reduce the scar tissue and restore pain-free motion. Facilitated stretching, when used appropriately with manual soft tissue therapy, can increase the likelihood of safely and effectively restoring pain-free motion to injured tissues.

Modifying Fibrotic Tissue to Reduce Pain and Restore Range of Motion

Scar tissue or adhesions can develop within and between muscles, fascia, and neural tissues. These adhesions can cause an array of problems, from minor periodic discomfort to severe progressive compensatory dysfunction and even nerve damage.

Scar tissue may develop because of acute trauma to the tissues or over time as repetitive stress injury. Although scar tissue formation is a normal response to injury, excessive scarring reduces function and contributes to chronic pain and limitation of movement.

Adhesions are nonfunctional cross-links between fibers within a muscle or between layers of muscle, in fascia, or in neural tissues. These cross-links prevent normal motion, and this limitation is often accompanied by pain. Adhesions can form as a result of postural stress, chronic hypertonicity in a muscle, or lack of motion.

The terms "adhesions" and "scar tissue" are often used interchangeably. In the following discussion we refer to these formations collectively as fibrotic tissue.

Admittedly, much of what follows is based on clinical experience and anecdotal evidence, not on controlled studies.

Many forms of manual soft tissue therapy are used to reduce the restriction and pain caused by fibrotic tissue. When facilitated stretching is added to the mix, better results can be achieved. This combination of stretching and soft tissue work is used only on chronic injuries and rarely with acute injuries. During the acute phase, we must be careful not to disrupt newly forming scar tissue. Stretching or deep soft tissue work is usually contraindicated until the scar tissue has matured.

Blending Soft Tissue Work and Facilitated Stretching

A typical treatment scenario for chronic injury begins with an evaluation of the range of motion (ROM) of the injured area, noting where pain is felt and at what point in the motion it begins. Soft tissue work is performed, if appropriate. This work is followed by facilitated stretching, within the pain-free ROM, to attempt to increase the pain-free range. Once the new limits of pain-free motion are achieved using facilitated stretching, a small amount of passive stretch is added to pinpoint the exact area where pain is felt in the stretched tissues. We theorize that this painful area is the site of fibrotic tissue and may be extremely small. Once this area is located, the passive stretch is released slightly until the client is once again at the pain-free end of range. Specific soft tissue techniques to release the fibrosis (such as transverse friction massage) can then be used on the exact site of the pain. This treatment is immediately followed by gentle active or passive movement to lengthen the treated tissue to a new pain-free range. Another round of facilitated stretching is then initiated. In most cases, the pain-free ROM increases again as a result of this combination of techniques.

Combining facilitated stretching and soft tissue therapy reduces fibrotic tissue more completely than either technique alone. Soft tissue therapies, such as deep transverse friction and pin-and-stretch techniques, have long been used to break down excessive scar tissue or to free adhesions from surrounding tissues, bone, or both. We hypothesize that the soft tissue work breaks free some of the fibrosis and that additional cross-links are released with the application of facilitated stretching immediately following. In a sense, the soft tissue work softens up the fibrotic tissue so that stretching is capable of "snapping" fibers that have not been released through the manual technique.

Releasing Fibrotic Tissue: Six Examples

Specific treatment scenarios may be helpful here. Remember, this combination of techniques is used only with chronic injuries, not acute ones.

Releasing the Scalenes

You're treating a patient with chronic pain and limited cervical ROM secondary to whiplash injuries sustained in an auto accident; specifically, when she laterally flexes to the right, she feels pain on the left side of her neck. She has been medically evaluated, and structural problems, such as a vertebral or disc-related cause for the pain, have been ruled out. This pain pattern, then, would indicate that pain is the result of injured soft tissues, probably the right scalenes. Treatment begins with general soft tissue work to release tension and warm up the muscles of the neck. Then, with the patient supine on the treatment table, ask her to laterally flex to the right as far as she can without pain. Use facilitated stretching for the left scalenes to try to increase her pain-free range in lateral flexion to the right (see the scalene stretch, p. 117).

Following this stretch, whether or not you've gained more ROM, laterally flex her to the right passively, just far enough for her to pinpoint the painful area that now limits her motion. Once it is located, release the passive stretch slightly so that she is once again in a position of comfort. Now, apply friction massage, or a similar technique, to release the fibrotic tissue causing the pain and limitation (figure 7.1). After this treatment, ask the client to actively move farther into pain-free lateral flexion to the right, or gently move her passively. She should be able to increase her pain-free range following the soft tissue treatment, though this is not always the case. At whatever her pain-free range is now, initiate another round of facilitated stretching to increase it further.

Releasing the Hamstrings

Another example of this treatment would involve a client with a chronic hamstring pull resulting in an inflammatory response and subsequent fibrotic tissue

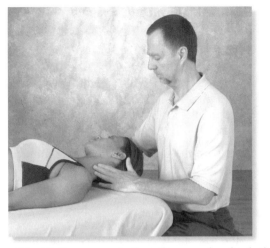

Figure 7.1 Friction massage to the scalene muscles after facilitated stretching.

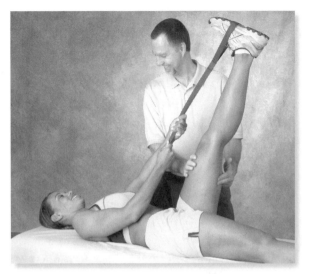

Figure 7.2 Friction massage to the hamstring muscles after facilitated stretching.

formation in the belly of the hamstrings. Examination reveals restricted flexibility in the hamstrings and pain at the site of the fibrotic tissue.

Typical treatment may consist of soft tissue work to the hamstrings, heat or ice, and self-directed stretching at home. If the client does not respond to this scenario, you can add facilitated stretching immediately following your soft tissue work.

In the supine position, have the stretcher actively flex her hip with the knee extended to the point where she feels the restriction. Perform several sets of facilitated stretching on the involved hamstring.

If you want to emphasize the medial hamstring more, use the spiral pattern for D2 flexion (see p. 79), which will focus the isometric effort and the subsequent stretch to the medial hamstring. To emphasize the lateral hamstrings, use D1 flexion (see p. 77). The exact position of the leg in these patterns can be fine-tuned to work directly through the line of restriction felt by the client.

After you've completed the stretching, you can once again employ specific soft tissue work to continue to release adhesions in the hamstrings. Stretch the hamstrings passively just to the point of pain or restriction so that the client can identify the exact site. Release the passive stretch slightly so that the client is once again in a position of comfort, and begin your specific soft tissue work (figure 7.2). Once that is completed, try again to increase the pain-free ROM using facilitated stretching.

Releasing the Hip, Side-Lying

The side-lying position provides excellent access for working on the hip abductors. The majority of clients we have treated over the years have had abductor involvement, no matter their primary complaint. Because the abductors act more as postural muscles than as prime movers, they can become extremely hypertonic, fibrotic, and tender to palpation, even though the client may not be experiencing any overt symptoms.

The side-lying position also allows easy access to the oblique abdominal muscles, the quadratus lumborum, and the latissimus dorsi. These muscles can all be involved when the client has "hip issues."

Position the client side-lying, hips stacked vertically, bottom leg flexed toward the chest, top leg hanging off the back of the treatment table. This is the same as the starting position for stretching the hip abductors (see p. 49). At this point, the client can usually pinpoint an area of slight to moderate discomfort in the hip abductor group. Try using a couple of rounds of stretching to reduce or eliminate this discomfort; then ask the client to identify any continuing sense of restriction or discomfort. Typically, the client will be able to isolate a very small area or point of restriction.

Apply some form of soft tissue work (like transverse friction) to the site of restriction for a minute or so; then check with the client to see if anything has changed (figure 7.3, p. 134). It's not uncommon to see a spontaneous improvement in ROM and for the client to report that the discomfort is now gone.

The client will also usually be able to identify a new area of discomfort, most often higher up on the iliac crest, along the attachment of the oblique abdominal muscles. You can continue to repeat the sequence of stretch and soft tissue work until you clear the entire area.

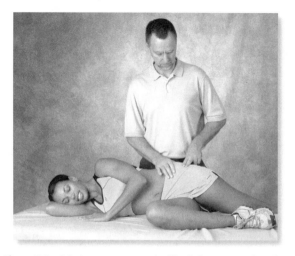

Figure 7.3 **Friction massage to the hip abductor muscles after facilitated stretching.**

Releasing the Piriformis, Prone

The piriformis is a lateral rotator of the hip. Successfully releasing the piriformis can be extremely rewarding for the therapist and the client because the pain associated with problems in this area can be quite debilitating. For instance, piriformis syndrome is a condition with symptoms that mimic sciatica. In this condition, the sciatic nerve is entrapped as it travels through the sciatic notch or as it courses through the posterior hip. "Nervy" pain is usually felt down the posterior thigh.

Piriformis also acts as a postural stabilizer. When hypertonic, it can alter the mechanics of sacral motion by causing an excessive shearing pressure on the sacroiliac (S-I) joint. This pressure often leads to pain and discomfort in the low back, S-I, or both.

Several techniques can be combined with facilitated stretching to help restore normal tone and texture to the piriformis and the other lateral rotators of the hip.

Prepare the piriformis for more focused work using any soft tissue technique to release tension and warm up the entire gluteal area. Perform a round or two of facilitated stretching. Then try one or more the following techniques.

Pin-and-Stretch Technique: Piriformis

1. With the client prone, stand at the affected side and ask the client to flex her knee to 90 degrees, then externally rotate the thigh to bring the lower leg across the midline as far as possible. Use your distal hand to lightly grasp the client's leg at the ankle. Your proximal hand will apply pressure to the piriformis during the application of this technique. A loose fist

is used for general contact (figure 7.4a); the thumb is used for more specific contact.

2. With the leg in the starting position just described, apply pressure to the piriformis with a loose fist and maintain that pressure while you passively rotate the thigh internally, that is, pull the foot and ankle toward you as far as possible.

3. Release the pressure on the piriformis, return the leg to the starting position, reapply pressure in a different place on the piriformis, and repeat.

4. Systematically work the whole piriformis, then the rest of the lateral rotators of the hip.

5. After the first round using a loose fist is completed, repeat, using a flat thumb for more specific contact (figure 7.4b).

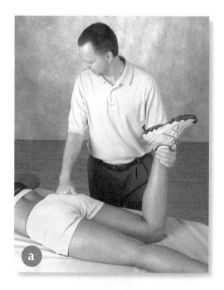

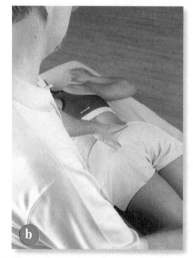

Figure 7.4 **Pin-and-stretch technique for the piriformis:** *(a)* **loose fist contact and** *(b)* **flat thumb contact.**

Transverse Friction Technique: Piriformis

1. Light friction work along the sacral border is especially effective when the piriformis has been softened with other techniques. Friction is applied across the grain of the muscle, using the thumb or fingers to rub against the lateral border of the sacrum (figure 7.5a).

2. Be certain that the friction work does not cause any numbness or tingling, since this indicates that you are frictioning right on the sciatic nerve.

3. Friction is also effective when applied at the insertion point on the greater trochanter (figure 7.5b).

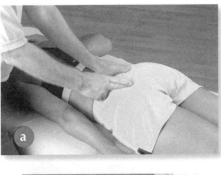

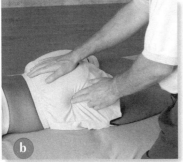

Figure 7.5   **Transverse friction for the piriformis:** *(a)* **along the sacral border and** *(b)* **at the attachment on the greater trochanter.**

Isolytic Contraction Technique: Piriformis

An isolytic contraction is an isotonic, eccentric contraction performed with the intent of stretching and breaking down fibrotic tissue (Chaitow 2001). It can be uncomfortable for the client, so proceed with caution to be sure you're not exceeding her tolerance level.

1. With the client prone, stand at the affected side and ask the client to flex her knee to 90 degrees, then externally rotate the thigh to bring the leg across the midline as far as possible. This shortens the piriformis. Use your distal hand to lightly grasp the client's leg at the ankle; your proximal hand stabilizes the pelvis (figure 7.6).

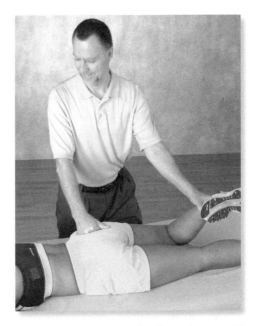

Figure 7.6   **Isolytic contraction for the piriformis. With each subsequent isolytic contraction, the client resists more strongly to recruit more muscle fibers.**

2. From this starting position, ask the client to lightly resist as you slowly pull the leg toward you, internally rotating the thigh as far as possible to lengthen the piriformis.

3. Repeat three times. In the beginning, the client's resistance should be minimal; then, with each subsequent isolytic contraction, the client resists more strongly to recruit more muscle fibers.

4. During each repetition, apply just enough counterforce to overcome the client's contraction. This activity should all be pain free.

Releasing the Subscapularis

The subscapularis is one of the four rotator cuff muscles and is responsible for medial rotation of the humerus. It also acts as a stabilizer for the humeral head in the glenoid fossa. When the subscapularis is not functioning optimally, it may allow the humerus to drift superiorly, creating impingement symptoms as the humerus rubs against the acromion.

Prepare the subscapularis for more focused work using any soft tissue technique to release tension and warm up the shoulder girdle. Perform a round or two of facilitated stretching (see p. 85). Then try the following technique.

Pin-and-Stretch Technique: Subscapularis

1. The client is supine. Standing near the client's head, flex and support the left humerus, holding the arm at the elbow with your right hand. Passively move the client's arm back toward the table (shoulder extension) to slacken the axillary tissues; gently palpate with your left hand (flat thumb or finger pads) anterior to the latissimus and teres major until you are on the anterior surface of the scapula, that is, in contact with the edge of the subscapularis (figure 7.7a). This contact may be uncomfortable for the client, but should not be painful.

2. Maintain mild to moderate pressure on the subscapularis as you slowly draw the left arm into flexion again, as far as is comfortable for the client (figure 7.7b).

3. Immediately reverse into extension and move your contact to a new place on the subscapularis, then draw the arm back into flexion.

4. Systematically release as much of the subscapularis as you can palpate.

Releasing the Serratus Anterior

When serratus anterior is hypertonic, it can cause the scapula to protract excessively, altering the mechanics of the shoulder joint. This hypertonicity also adds eccentric stress to the rhomboids, causing them to feel sore and tight.

Adding specific soft tissue work to facilitated stretching will enable you to more effectively normalize the tone and texture of this muscle. Prepare the serratus for more focused work using any soft tissue technique

to release tension and warm up the shoulder girdle. Perform a round or two of facilitated stretching (see p. 86). Then try the following technique.

Transverse Friction Technique: Serratus Anterior

1. With the client prone, "wing" the scapula using whatever technique you're comfortable with. We prefer to have the client's arm resting at her side so that we can use a hand under the anterior shoulder to lift and retract the scapula.

2. With the opposite hand, palpate the anterior surface along the medial border of the scapula to locate the serratus anterior. Apply transverse friction strokes along this attachment of the muscle (figure 7.8a).

3. Maintaining the scapula in the winged position, use a pincer palpation to work your way into the wad of serratus on the anterior scapula at its inferior angle.

4. Once there, use a sawing type of transverse friction to affect the muscle (figure 7.8b).

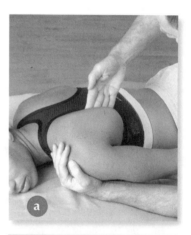

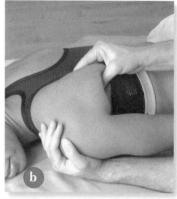

Figure 7.8 Transverse friction for the serratus anterior: (a) along the medial border of the scapula and (b) applying friction using a pincer grip of the muscle.

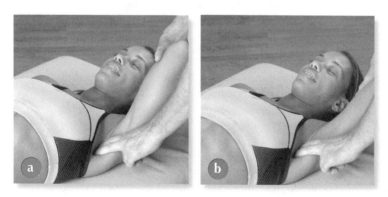

Figure 7.7 Pin-and-stretch technique for the subscapularis: (a) initial contact and (b) passive stretch of the pinned muscle.

CHAPTER 8

Stretching Routines for Specific Activities

Stretching is more effective if your muscles are warmed up first. If you are using these stretches prior to exercise, we suggest 5 to 15 minutes of light activity to warm up before you stretch.

We have a natural tendency to spend more time stretching the first arm, leg, or area; and because it's natural to stretch the easy side first, the tighter side usually gets less attention. To counteract this, focus on stretching your tighter side first. This will help you gain overall balanced flexibility.

Regular practice is the most important part of any flexibility program.

Perform two to three rounds of stretching for each muscle, which will take 30 to 45 seconds total.

Each sport places differing demands on the body in terms of strength and flexibility. The best approach to enhancing performance and staying injury free is to develop balanced strength and flexibility throughout the body. The following routines cover the primary muscle groups involved in particular activities. To a certain extent, the grouping of stretches is arbitrary, and you may decide you need to add or subtract stretches to fit your particular situation.

RUNNING

(11 self-stretches on each side, approximate time to complete: 10-12 minutes)

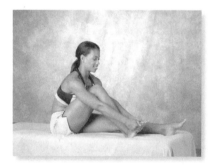

1 **Gluteus Maximus**
Page 42

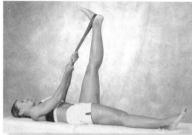

2 **Hamstrings**
Page 41

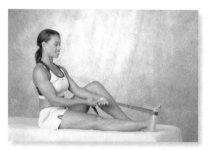

3 **Gastrocnemius**
Page 63

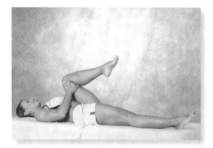

4 **Soleus**
Page 64

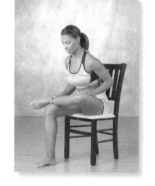

5 **Piriformis**
Page 46

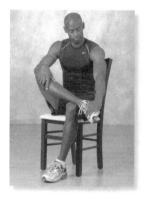

6 **Tibialis Anterior**
Page 69

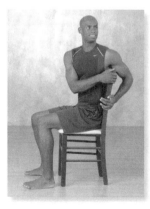

7 **Trunk Rotators**
Page 123

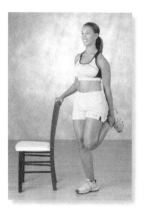

8 **Quadriceps**
Page 57

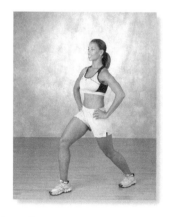

9 **Psoas**
Page 60

RUNNING

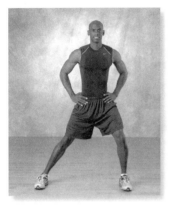

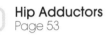 **Hip Adductors**
Page 53

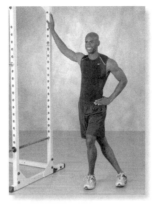

11 **Hip Abductors**
Page 50

THROWING AND RACKET SPORTS

(18 self-stretches on each side, approximate time to complete: 15-18 minutes)

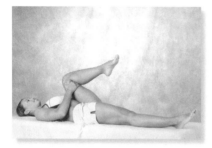

1 Gluteus Maximus
Page 42

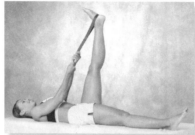

2 Hamstrings
Page 41

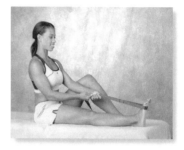

3 Gastrocnemius
Page 63

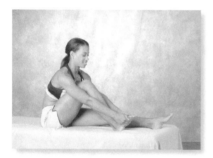

4 Soleus
Page 64

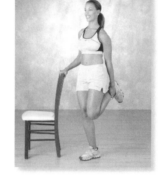

5 Quadriceps
Page 57

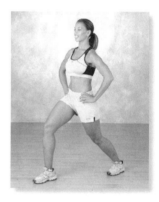

6 Psoas
Page 60

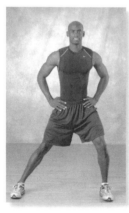

7 Hip Adductors
Page 53

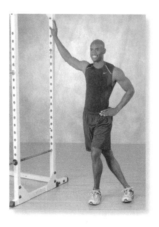

8 Hip Abductors
Page 50

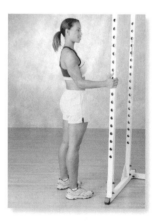

9 Subscapularis
Page 85

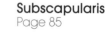

THROWING AND RACKET SPORTS

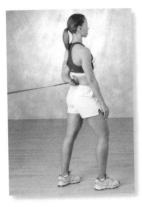

10 **Infraspinatus**
Page 86

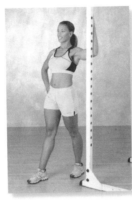

11 **Pectoralis Major**
Page 92

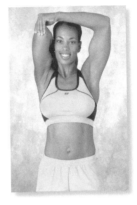

12 **Triceps**
Page 94

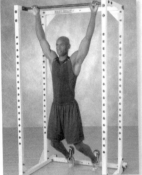

13 **Latissimus Dorsi**
Page 125

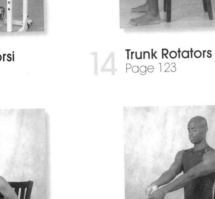

14 **Trunk Rotators**
Page 123

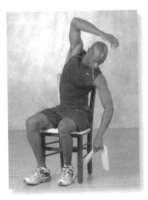

15 **Quadratus Lumborum**
Page 125

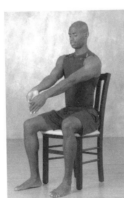

16 **Piriformis**
Page 46

17 **Wrist Extensors**
Page 99

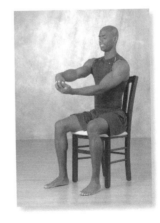

18 **Wrist Flexors**
Page 100

CYCLING

(14 self-stretches on each side, approximate time to complete: 15-18 minutes)

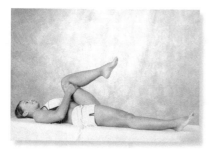

1 **Gluteus Maximus**
Page 42

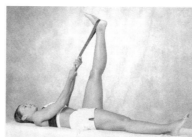

2 **Hamstrings**
Page 41

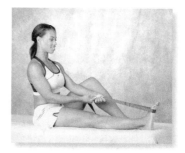

3 **Gastrocnemius**
Page 63

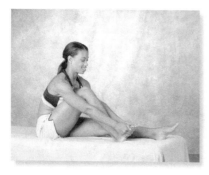

4 **Soleus**
Page 64

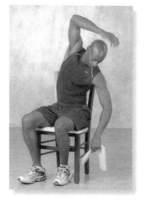

5 **Quadratus Lumborum**
Page 124

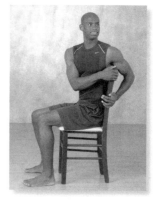

6 **Trunk Rotators**
Page 123

CYCLING

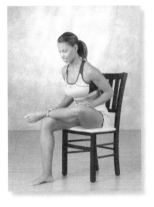

7 **Piriformis**
Page 46

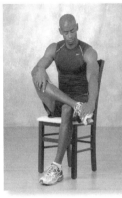

8 **Tibialis Anterior**
Page 69

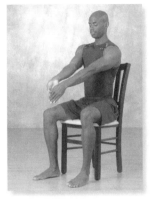

9 **Wrist Flexors**
Page 99

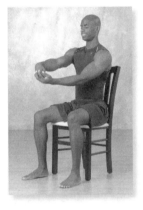

10 **Wrist Extensors**
Page 100

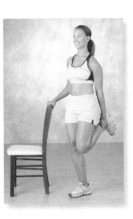

11 **Quadriceps**
Page 57

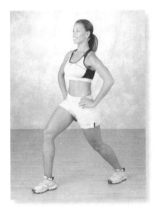

12 **Psoas**
Page 60

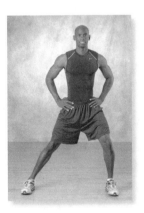

13 **Hip Adductors**
Page 53

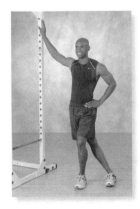

14 **Hip Abductors**
Page 50

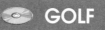 **GOLF**

(15 self-stretches on each side, approximate time to complete: 16-20 minutes)

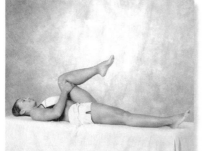

1 **Gluteus Maximus**
Page 42

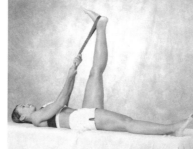

2 **Hamstrings**
Page 41

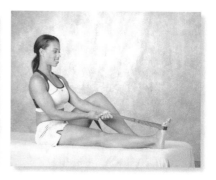

3 **Gastrocnemius**
Page 63

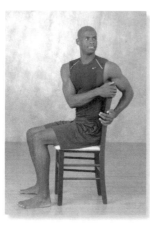

4 **Trunk Rotators**
Page 122

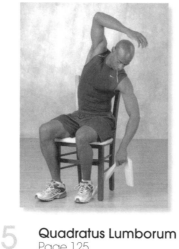

5 **Quadratus Lumborum**
Page 125

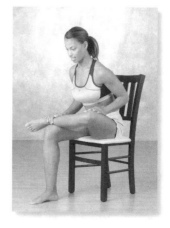

6 **Piriformis**
Page 46

GOLF

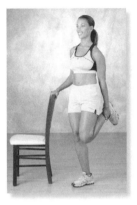

7 **Quadriceps**
Page 57

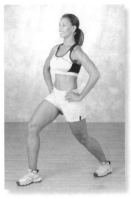

8 **Psoas**
Page 60

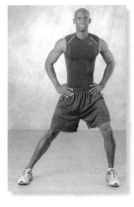

9 **Hip Adductors**
Page 53

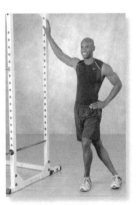

10 **Hip Abductors**
Page 50

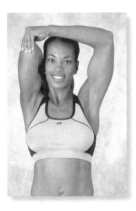

11 **Triceps**
Page 94

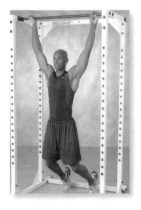

12 **Latissimus Dorsi**
Page 126

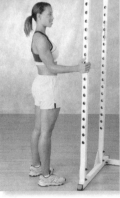

13 **Subscapularis**
Page 85

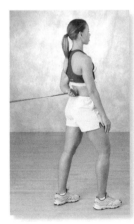

14 **Infraspinatus**
Page 86

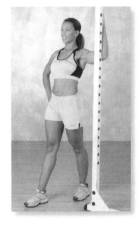

15 **Pectoralis Major**
Page 92

SWIMMING

(16 self-stretches on each side, approximate time to complete: 16-20 minutes)

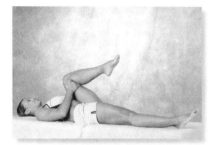

1 **Gluteus Maximus**
Page 42

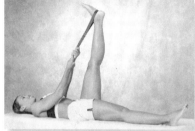

2 **Hamstrings**
Page 41

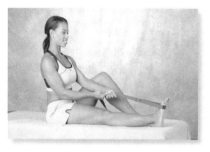

3 **Gastrocnemius**
Page 63

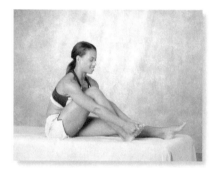

4 **Soleus**
Page 64

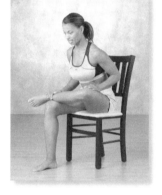

5 **Piriformis**
Page 46

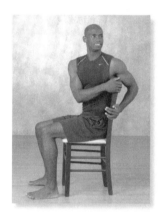

6 **Trunk Rotators**
Page 123

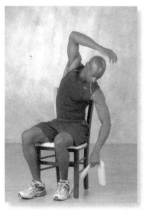

7 **Quadratus Lumborum**
Page 125

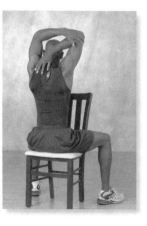

8 **Latissimus Dorsi**
Page 126

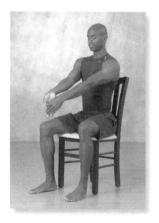

9 **Wrist Flexors**
Page 15

SWIMMING

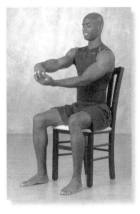

10 **Wrist Extensors**
Page 100

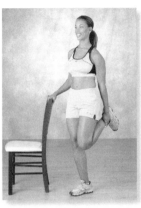

11 **Quadriceps**
Page 57

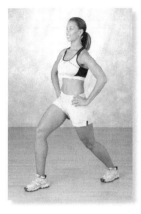

12 **Psoas**
Page 60

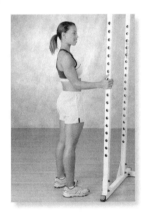

13 **Subscapularis**
Page 85

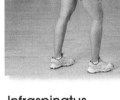

14 **Infraspinatus**
Page 86

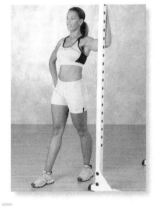

15 **Pectoralis Major**
Page 92

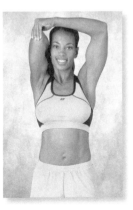

16 **Triceps**
Page 94

EVERYDAY SEQUENCE

(14 self-stretches on each side, approximate time to complete: 15-18 minutes)

The stretches grouped here are an excellent way to begin and end the day. In the morning, they will help energize and limber your body. When done in the evening, they will help you unwind and shed the day's tensions.

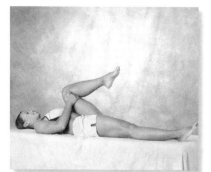
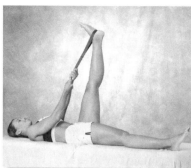
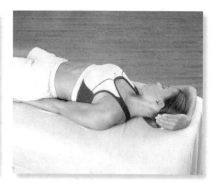
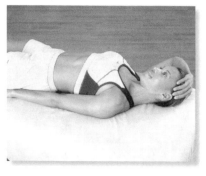
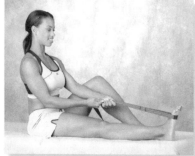
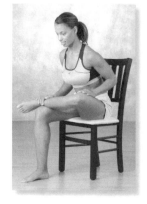

1 **Gluteus Maximus**
Page 42

2 **Hamstrings**
Page 41

3 **Upper Trapezius**
Page 115

4 **Scalenes**
Page 116

5 **Gastrocnemius**
Page 63

6 **Piriformis**
Page 46

EVERYDAY SEQUENCE

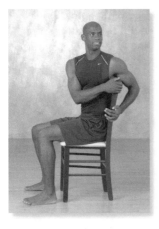

7 **Trunk Rotators**
Page 123

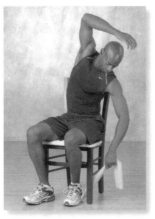

8 **Quadratus Lumborum**
Page 125s

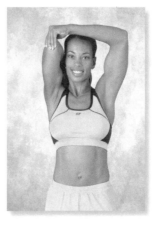

9 **Triceps**
Page 94

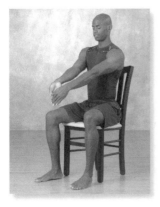

10 **Wrist Flexors**
Page 99

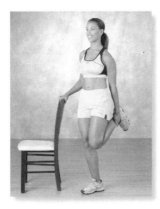

11 **Quadriceps**
Page 57

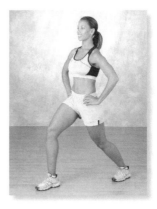

12 **Psoas**
Page 60

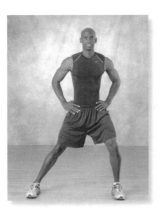

13 **Hip Adductors**
Page 53

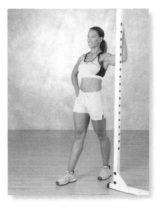

14 **Pectoralis Major**
Page 92

RUSTY HINGES

(14 self-stretches on each side, approximate time to complete: 15-18 minutes)

As we age, we tend to lose flexibility, which causes us to move with more difficulty. This begins a vicious downward spiral that can lead to severely restricted range of motion, loss of strength, and poor balance. These stretches are excellent for maintaining or restoring joint mobility, muscular strength, and coordination. They may also help to relieve pain.

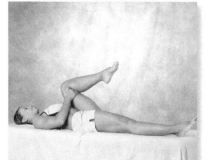

1 **Gluteus Maximus**
Page 42

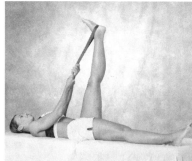

2 **Hamstrings**
Page 41

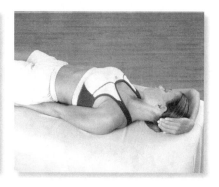

3 **Upper Trapezius**
Page 115

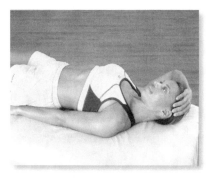

4 **Scalenes**
Page 117

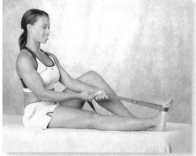

5 **Gastrocnemius**
Page 63

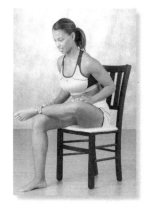

6 **Piriformis**
Page 46

RUSTY HINGES

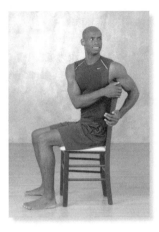

7 **Trunk Rotators**
Page 123

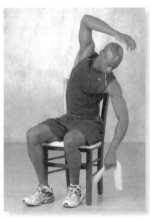

8 **Quadratus Lumborum**
Page 125

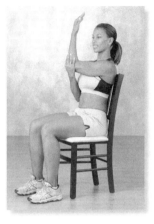

9 **Rhomboids**
Page 88

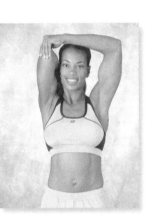

10 **Triceps**
Page 94

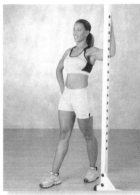

11 **Pectoralis Major**
Page 92

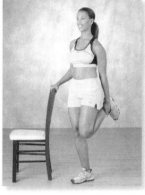

12 **Quadriceps**
Page 57

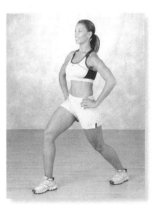

13 **Psoas**
Page 60

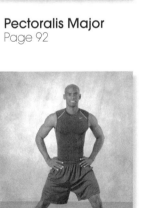

14 **Hip Adductors**
Page 53

Routines for Common Soft Tissue Injuries

With Dave Charland, ATC, PT

This chapter illustrates how facilitated stretching can be incorporated into a practical approach to treating some of the more common injuries that most people experience at some time in their lives. Stretching not only feels good; it can also help improve function and prevent or help resolve some painful conditions.

This chapter offers some self-help remedies that may alleviate or at least reduce the "nagging," uncomfortable conditions that so many just learn to live with.

We share 40+ years of combined experience dealing with painful conditions in our clients and patients. We've included easy-to-follow exercise programs that have worked for us over the years. These programs are effective for treating yourself, on your own, at home or in the gym.

Nevertheless, we recommend consulting with your health care provider before starting on any exercise program.

Caring for Acute and Chronic Injuries

Let's start by summarizing the basics for treating any acute soft tissue injury. An acute strain or injury is one that happened less than 30 days ago, or one in which active inflammation is present.

Acute injuries are best treated using the RICE principle (Rest, Ice, Compression, Elevation). The body, when newly injured, responds with an inflammatory reaction, which is normal and good; but the swelling and inflammation, if unchecked, may interfere with healing. RICE aids in controlling the inflammatory response and with the overall healing process.

In the acute stage, injuries should be treated conservatively, with gentle stretching and pain-free exercise.

For the more chronic or nagging injuries, it may be helpful to warm up the area first to prepare the tissues for the stretching and exercise activity. Those old troublesome areas respond well to a moist heat pack, hot shower, hot tub, or even easy bike riding or jogging. These activities all help to get the blood flowing, lubricate the joints, and release endorphins, creating pain relief and more limber muscles.

In the following pages, we identify the injuries, suggest appropriate stretching and strengthening activities, and offer alternative activities, precautions, or both. For quicker reference, we group and separate upper body and lower body conditions.

Focusing on Upper Body Conditions

We discuss neck, shoulder, elbow, and wrist problems in this section. In cases where the same exercise program is recommended for more than one of these conditions, we describe the conditions first, then list the exercise program.

Painful Trigger Points in the Neck and Shoulder Area

Trigger points can cause several types of pain, but the most common are usually described by patients as a "deep ache" or as "numbing, tingling, shooting" pain.

Some other conditions that may cause similar symptoms are torticollis (wryneck), cervical strain or sprain, and cervicalgia. These should all be ruled out before you engage in the following activities.

The reasons trigger points develop are numerous and may all happen at once. They include (but aren't limited to) sleeping in the wrong position, lifting something improperly, turning toward something and getting bumped, stress, driving, working on the computer, or sitting at a desk for a long period of time.

After identifying the problem, your physician has several choices for care, which may include rest, nonsteroidal anti-inflammatory medications, trigger point injections, cervical collar, physical therapy, massage therapy, or acupuncture.

The condition may be further complicated by other factors such as spinal instability, herniated disc, or arthritis. These factors may prevent you from resolving your pain with a home exercise program. However, these exercises, if done correctly, will not cause further injury to your neck and shoulders.

Obviously, if your condition is worsening over time while you are trying these exercises, you should see your medical provider.

STRETCHES

The following activities should not cause pain, but should allow for gentle increases in mobility and greater use of the head and neck.

1. Upper trapezius, page 114-115
2. Scalenes, page 116-117
3. Sternocleidomastoid, page 115
4. Levator scapulae, page 118-119
5. Suboccipitals, page 118

STRENGTHENING EXERCISES

These activities can be made more challenging if the use of an elastic band or tubing is added. Resistance should be added only when the joint can be moved without pain.

Shoulder Shrugs (Standing or Sitting)

Put your elbows by your side with elbows bent. Raise your shoulders upward and be sure to squeeze the shoulder blades together (figure 9.1). Repeat 8 to 10 times.

Scapula Pinches

Squeeze your shoulder blades together, aiming the right blade toward the left back pocket and the left blade toward the right back pocket (figure 9.2). Repeat 8 to 10 times.

Isometrics of the Neck (Standing or Sitting)

Flexion

Put your hands in front of your head and press your head forward gently, not allowing any neck movement. Hold for 6 seconds, then relax. Repeat five times (figure 9.3).

Extension

Put your hands in back of your head and press your head backward gently, not allowing any neck movement. Hold for 6 seconds, then relax. Repeat five times (figure 9.4).

Lateral Flexion

Right: Put your hand on the right side of your head and press your head to the right gently (ear toward shoulder), not allowing any neck movement. Hold for 6 seconds, then relax. Repeat five times (figure 9.5). Repeat on left side.

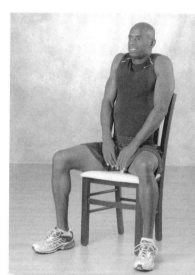

Figure 9.1   **Shoulder shrugs.**

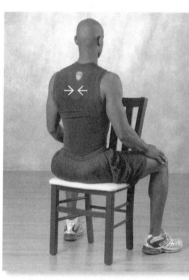

Figure 9.2   **Scapula pinches.**

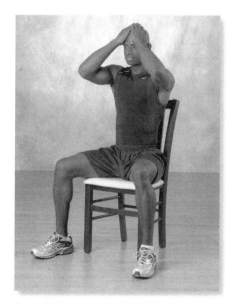

Figure 9.3   **Isometric neck flexion.**

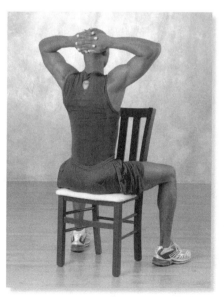

Figure 9.4   **Isometric neck extension.**

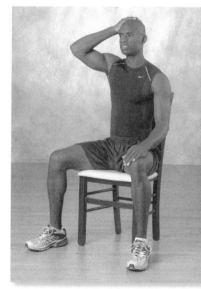

Figure 9.5   **Isometric neck lateral flexion.**

UPPER BODY CONDITIONS

Rotation

Right: Put your hand on the right side of your head and look to the right with your eyes only. Turn your head into your hand gently, not allowing any neck movement. Hold for 6 seconds, then relax. Repeat five times (figure 9.6). Repeat on left side.

Shoulder Rotation

Internal Rotation

Using an elastic band that has been attached to the door or other fixed object, hold the other end in your right hand while standing or sitting with your right side to the wall. Bend your elbow to form a right angle, and pull the band across your body so your hand moves toward your stomach, then slowly return to the start. Repeat 8 to 10 times. Adjust the resistance by taking up or allowing more slack in the band. Repeat on the left side (figure 9.7).

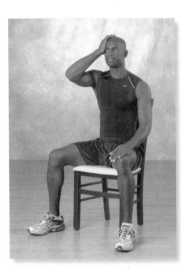

Figure 9.6 **Isometric neck rotation.**

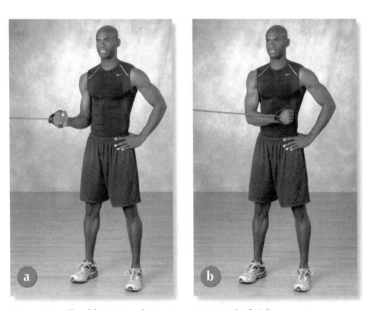

Figure 9.7 **Shoulder internal rotation:** *(a)* **start,** *(b)* **finish.**

External Rotation (Bilateral)

Using both hands, grasp an elastic band at each end while standing or sitting. Bend your elbows so that each forms a right angle, keep them tight against your side, and pull the band outward. Repeat 8 to 10 times. Adjust the resistance by taking up or allowing more slack in the band (figure 9.8).

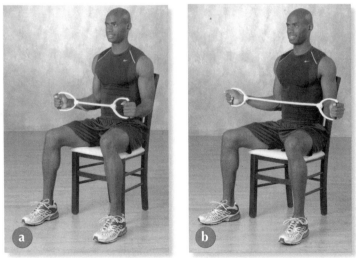

Figure 9.8 **Shoulder external rotation:** *(a)* **start,** *(b)* **finish.**

PNF Patterns

Diagonal Two (Sword)

(Repeat each motion 8 to 10 times; may be done simultaneously.)

Stand with a light weight in your right hand (or use a cuff weight if that's easier). Starting with your palm down and across your body, raise your arm upward overhead and outward and rotate your palm upward in a diagonal direction, as if raising a sword overhead (figure 9.9). Reverse direction and repeat. Repeat the D2 pattern with the left arm, or do the two motions simultaneously. See figure 3.4*b* on page 23 for other end of pattern.

Diagonal One (Seat Belt)

(Repeat each motion 8 to 10 times; may be done simultaneously.)

Stand with a light weight in your right hand (or use a cuff weight if that's easier). Starting with your palm facing back and your arm out and behind you (figure 9.10), raise your arm forward, upward, and across your body overhead in a diagonal direction, as if grabbing a seat belt. Reverse direction and repeat. Repeat the D1 pattern with the left arm, or do the two simultaneously. See figure 3.3*b*, p. 22 for the other end of the pattern.

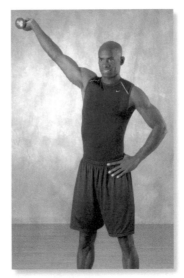

Figure 9.9 Diagonal two pattern with weight. End of draw sword motion.

SUPPLEMENTAL ACTIVITIES

1. Perform posture reinforcements (sitting up straight and slouching).
2. For acute injuries, apply ice first and then move gently. For chronic injuries, apply heat before doing activity.

PRECAUTIONS

1. Avoid circles with your neck.
2. Consider using a special pillow for sleeping.
3. Avoid sleeping with a breeze directly on your neck.

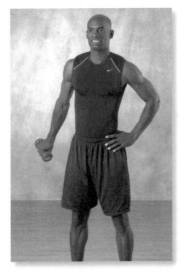

Figure 9.10 Diagonal one pattern with weight (seat belt).

Bursitis or Tendinitis in the Shoulder

Bursitis is inflammation and swelling of the bursa, a small sac of synovial fluid that is designed to cushion and protect the shoulder. Tendinitis is inflammation and swelling of one or more tendons around the shoulder.

Some common diagnoses are subacromial bursitis, rotator cuff tendinitis, biceps tendinitis, and impingement syndrome. Most of these conditions are caused by starting a new activity or overdoing an activity in a relatively short period of time. Once inflamed, shoulders normally take a long time to settle down because the shoulder is the most unstable joint in the body.

After identifying the problem, your physician has several choices for care, which may include rest, nonsteroidal anti-inflammatory medications, massage therapy, cortisone injection, physical therapy, or even surgery.

The condition may be further complicated by other factors such as instability, cartilage damage, or bone spurs. These factors may prevent you from resolving your pain with a home exercise program, but these exercises, if done correctly, will not cause you further injury.

Obviously, if your condition is worsening over time while you are trying these exercises, you should see your medical provider.

STRETCHES

The following activities should not cause pain, but should allow for gentle increases in mobility and greater use of the arms.

1. Pectoralis major, page 92
2. Subscapularis, page 85
3. Infraspinatus, pages 85-86
4. Latissimus dorsi, pages 125-126

STRENGTHENING EXERCISES

These activities can be made more challenging with the addition of use of an elastic band, tubing, or light cuff weights. Resistance should be added only when the joint can be moved without pain.

Scapula Pinches (for Lower Trapezius)

Standing or sitting, squeeze your shoulder blades together and toward each opposite back pocket. Repeat 8 to 10 times (see figure 9.2, p. 155).

Modified Seated Rows (for Rhomboids)

Standing or sitting, grasp the elastic band by each end after attaching it at elbow height to a door or other fixed object. Keep your arms straight and gently pull back by squeezing your shoulder blades together. Repeat 8 to 10 times. Adjust the resistance by taking up or allowing more slack in the band (figure 9.11).

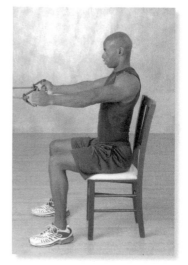

Figure 9.11 Modified seated rows (for rhomboids).

Rotator Cuff

Standing or sitting, hold your straight arms out in front at shoulder height, with thumbs pointing toward each other. Move your arms outward to 45 degrees and turn your thumbs down, and lower. Repeat 8 to 10 times (figure 9.12).

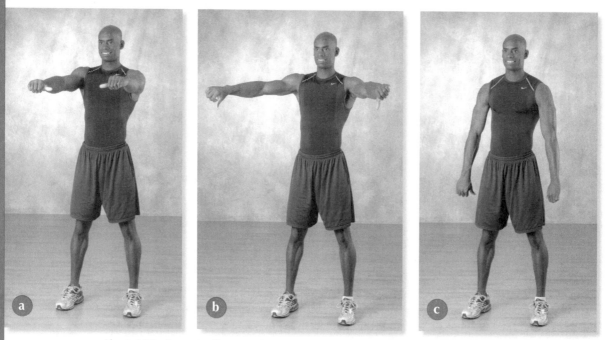

Figure 9.12 **Rotator cuff:** (a) **starting position,** (b) **middle position,** and (c) **end position.**

Deltoids

Anterior: Standing or sitting, straighten your arms; then raise them in front to shoulder height with your palms down, and lower them back down (figure 9.13*a*).

Middle: Standing or sitting, bend your elbows to 90 degrees; then raise them to the side and lower them back down (figure 9.13*b*).

Posterior: Lying on your stomach, raise your arms backward, with arms straight and palms facing the body, and lower them back down (figure 9.13*c*).

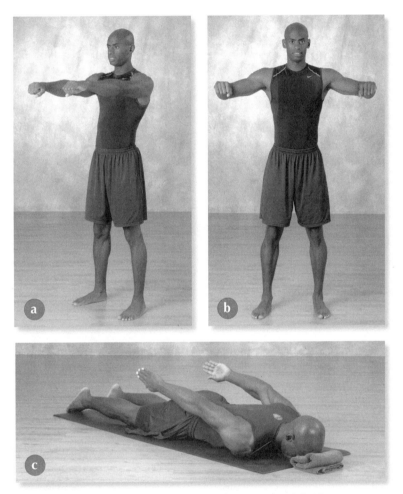

Figure 9.13 *(a)* **Anterior deltoids,** *(b)* **middle deltoids, and** *(c)* **posterior deltoids.**

PNF Patterns

Diagonal Two (Sword)
(Repeat each motion 8 to 10 times; may be done simultaneously.)

Stand with a light weight in your right hand (or use a cuff weight if that's easier). Starting with the palm down and across the body, raise your arm upward overhead and outward and rotate your palm upward in a diagonal direction, as if raising a sword overhead (see figure 9.9 on p. 157). Reverse direction and repeat. Repeat the D2 pattern with the left arm, or do both simultaneously.

Diagonal One (Seat Belt)
(Repeat each motion 8 to 10 times; may be done simultaneously.)

Stand with a light weight in your right hand (or use a cuff weight if it's easier). Start with your palm facing back and your arm out and behind you; raise the arm forward, upward, and across the body overhead in a diagonal direction as if grabbing a seat belt (see figure 9.10 on p. 155). Reverse direction and repeat. Repeat the D1 pattern with the left arm, or do both simultaneously.

SUPPLEMENTAL ACTIVITIES

1. Perform any back exercises.
2. Apply ice to the affected area frequently to help control inflammation and pain.

PRECAUTIONS

1. Avoid overhead activities.
2. Stop doing the bench press or military press.

Tennis Elbow

Tennis elbow is usually caused by repetitive stress that results in chronic strain and inflammation at the outer elbow.

Some common diagnoses are lateral epicondylitis, extensor tendinitis, elbow bursitis or tendinitis, and painful elbow. Most of these injuries are related to gripping or squeezing during bending and straightening of the elbow.

After identifying the problem, your physician has several choices for care, which may include rest, nonsteroidal anti-inflammatory medications, massage therapy, cortisone injection, straps or braces, physical therapy, or, as a last resort, surgery.

The difficulty with the resolution of this injury is the repetitive nature of everyday activities that continue to inflame this area. The condition may be further complicated by other factors such as instability or cartilage damage. These factors may prevent you from resolving your pain with a home exercise program. These exercises, if done correctly, will not cause you further injury and should improve your symptoms, even if they don't resolve them completely.

Carpal Tunnel Syndrome

Symptoms may include aching and numbness in the hands; difficulty grasping or holding on to objects; dropping things; or pain in the palm, forearm, or fingers (or more than one of these).

Some common diagnoses are cumulative trauma disorder, repetitive motion syndrome, multiple crush injury, and wrist sprain or strain. The causes for carpal tunnel syndrome are numerous and may be a combination of repetitive motion, especially keyboard use; other physical activity, like tightly holding on to a racket, club, bat, or other object; sleeping in the wrong position (with arms above your head or under you); lifting incorrectly; and stress.

After identifying the problem, your physician has several choices for care, which may include rest, nonsteroidal anti-inflammatory medications, trigger point injections, braces, splints, casts, massage therapy, physical therapy, acupuncture, or, as a last resort, surgery.

The condition may be further complicated by other factors such as thoracic outlet syndrome, poor postural alignment from tight muscles, joint instability, or malaligned joints. These factors may prevent you from resolving your pain with a home exercise program. These exercises, if done correctly, will not cause further injury to your wrists, hands, or fingers.

Obviously, if your condition is worsening over time while you are trying these exercises, stop them immediately and see your medical provider.

STRETCHES

These activities should not cause pain, but should allow for gentle increases in mobility and greater use of the elbow or arm (or both).

1. Wrist and finger flexors, page 99
2. Wrist and finger extensors, page 100

3. Biceps, page 93

4. Triceps, page 94

5. Forearm pronators and supinators, pages 101-102

STRENGTHENING EXERCISES

You can make these activities more challenging by adding the use of an elastic band or tubing. Resistance should be added only when the joint can be moved without increased pain.

Wrist Curls, Palm Up and Down

With a light weight in your hand, palm up, curl your wrist, bringing your fist toward you (flexion). With the palm down, bend the wrist backward, bringing the knuckles toward you (extension). Do a set of 8 to 10 for each (figure 9.14, *a & b*).

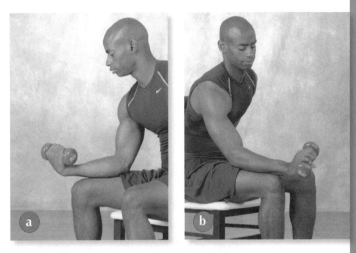

Figure 9.14   *(a)* **Wrist flexion.** *(b)* **Wrist extension.**

Radial Deviation

With your thumb pointing upward, bend your wrist upward, thumb toward you. Repeat 8 to 10 times (figure 9.15).

Ulnar Deviation

While standing, bend your wrist toward your little finger. Repeat 8 to 10 times (figure 9.16).

Finger Extension

Use a medium-size rubber band. Put it around the end of the fingers and your thumb and bring them apart. Repeat 8 to 10 times (figure 9.17).

PNF Patterns

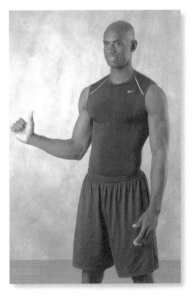

Figure 9.15   **Radial deviation.**

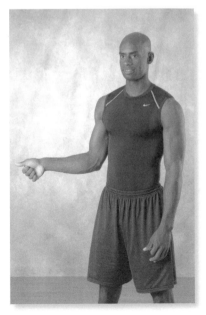

Figure 9.16   **Ulnar deviation.**

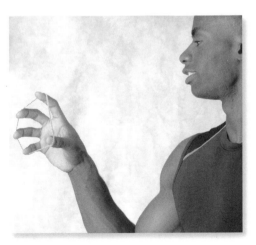

Figure 9.17   **Finger extension.**

UPPER BODY CONDITIONS

(Repeat 8 to 10 times; may be done on both sides simultaneously.)

Sit with a weight in your right hand. Start with your arm straight, palm facing down and away. Bend your elbow, rotating the palm up and out. Reverse the motion by rotating the palm down and out while straightening the arm (figure 9.18, *a* & *b*). Repeat 8 to 10 times. Do both sides.

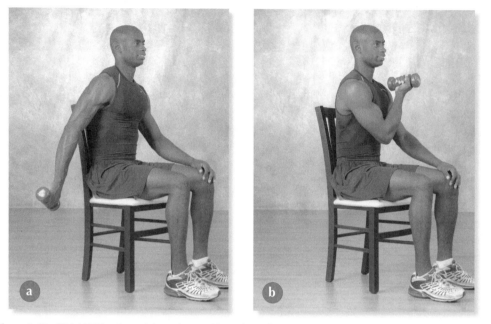

Figure 9.18   **Wrist PNF pattern:** *(a)* **starting position,** *(b)* **ending position.**

SUPPLEMENTAL ACTIVITIES

1. Isometric ball squeezes: Squeeze a sponge or a racquetball.
2. Putty exercises: Using putty or clay, squeeze, press into the putty with the fingers, pinch, and pull apart.
3. Ice massage.

PRECAUTIONS

1. Avoid heavy gripping.
2. Use a tennis elbow support or strap for a short time to reduce the pull on the extensor muscles.

Focusing on Lower Body Conditions

In this section we discuss hip, leg, and foot problems. Where the same exercise program is recommended for more than one of these conditions, we describe the conditions first, then list the exercise program.

Piriformis Syndrome

Piriformis syndrome is usually characterized by pain in the buttock area that radiates down the back of the thigh, sometimes all the way to the foot. The radiating pain is caused by irritation of the sciatic nerve as it runs through the buttock. This condition can be difficult to diagnose because the symptoms are similar to those for other conditions. This injury can also be confused with low back or hip conditions that radiate pain from the buttocks around to the front of the thigh.

Some other possible diagnoses are sciatica, buttocks pain, lumbago, gluteal strain, sacroiliac sprain or strain, and sacroiliac dysfunction.

After identifying the problem, your physician has several choices for care, which may include rest, nonsteroidal anti-inflammatory medications, cortisone injection, hip pads, physical therapy, or acupuncture.

The causes of piriformis syndrome are varied. They include (but aren't limited to) anatomical imbalances, lifting something improperly, turning toward something while bending at the hips, strenuous hiking or running, and sitting for long periods (especially on something like a wallet).

The condition may be further complicated by other factors such as instability, poor spinal alignment from tight muscles, or joint dysfunction. These factors may prevent you from resolving your pain with a home exercise program. However, these exercises, if done correctly, will not cause further injury to your hip, back, or buttocks and should improve your symptoms, even if they don't resolve them completely.

Trochanteric Bursitis

This condition is an inflammation of the bursa sac at the greater trochanter, the bony prominence commonly thought of as the outer hip. Symptoms are generally limited to the trochanter area and may include pain even during rest.

Some other common names for this condition are hip pain, hip pointer, hip sprain or strain, lateral hip pain, and hip or thigh myalgia.

After identifying the problem, your physician has several choices for care, which may include rest, nonsteroidal anti-inflammatory medications, cortisone injection, hip pads, physical therapy, or acupuncture.

The causes of trochanteric bursitis are numerous. They include (but aren't limited to) sleeping in the wrong position; lifting something improperly; getting bumped or bumping into something (for example, as you close a car door with your hip when your hands are full); prolonged bending from the hips; and sitting and working at a computer or at a desk for a long period of time, possibly in a tight chair.

This condition may be further complicated by other factors such as joint instability or poor spinal alignment from tight muscles. These factors may prevent you from resolving your pain with a home exercise program. However, these exercises, if done correctly, will not cause further injury to your hip and should improve your symptoms, even if they don't resolve them completely.

If your condition is worsening over time while you are trying these exercises, you should stop them and see your medical provider.

LOWER BODY CONDITIONS

STRETCHES

These activities should not cause pain, but should allow for gentle increases in mobility and greater use of your hips and back.

STRENGTHENING EXERCISES

You can make these activities more challenging by adding the use of an elastic band or tubing or light weights. Resistance should be added only when the joint can be moved without increased pain.

Open Chain (Non-Weight Bearing)

Knee Flexion, Sitting, to Strengthen Quads and Psoas

Sitting up straight in a chair, bend your knee back with the heel under the chair, then straighten out the leg while tightening your thigh (figure 9.19, a & b). Repeat 8 to 10 times on each side.

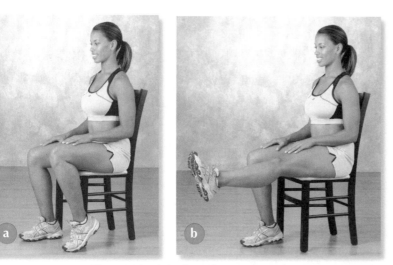

Figure 9.19   **Sitting knee flexion-extension:** *(a)* **start,** *(b)* **finish.**

Hip Flexion, Sitting, to Strengthen Psoas (Marching in Place)

Sitting up straight in a chair, keeping your knees bent, raise your knee up, bending at the hip. Alternate legs (figure 9.20). Repeat 8 to 10 times on each side.

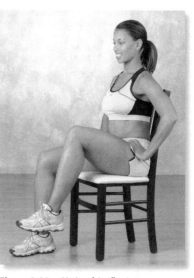

Figure 9.20   **Sitting hip flexion.**

Straight Leg Raises—All Four Directions

Flexion

Lie on your back with both legs straight out or your left knee bent, with the left foot flat on the mat. Lift your right leg upward, hold (1-2 seconds), and lower slowly. Breathe normally and repeat 8 to 10 times. Change leg positions and repeat on the other side (figure 9.21).

Abduction-Adduction

Lie on your back with your left leg straight out and your right knee bent, with the right foot flat on the mat. Lift your left leg up and bring it out away from your midline, hold (1-2 seconds), and slowly pull back in toward the middle. Breathe normally and repeat 8 to 10 times. Change leg positions and repeat on the other side (figure 9.22).

Extension

Lie on your stomach, with your legs out straight. Lift your right leg upward, keeping it straight, hold (1-2 seconds), and lower slowly. Breathe normally and repeat 8 to 10 times. Repeat on the other side (figure 9.23).

Hip-Knee-Ankle Combination PNF Diagonals

You may use ankle weights to give a little resistance for either direction of movement.

Diagonal One

Lie on your back. Bring your left leg upward, bend the knee to bring the heel to your buttock, flex the ankle so the toes are pointing toward your head, and aim your left knee toward the opposite shoulder. Then lower the leg while straightening the knee, pointing the toes down, and bringing the leg outward to the side. This movement will be a combination of up and across and down and out (figure 9.24, a-c). Repeat 8 to 10 times, then change sides and repeat.

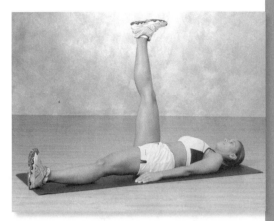

Figure 9.21 Leg raises, flexion.

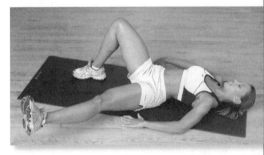

Figure 9.22 Leg raises, abduction-adduction.

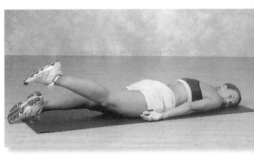

Figure 9.23 Leg raises, extension.

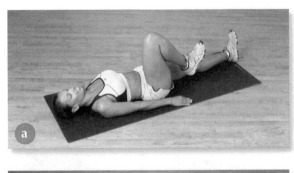

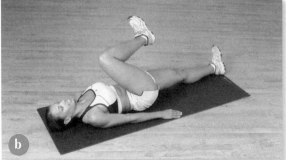

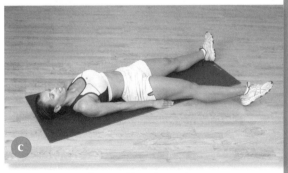

Figure 9.24 Hip-knee-ankle, Diagonal one: *(a)* heel to buttock, *(b)* knee toward shoulder, and *(c)* toes down and out.

LOWER BODY CONDITIONS

Diagonal Two

Lie on your back. Bring your right leg upward, bend the knee to bring the heel to your buttock, flex the ankle so the toes are pointing toward your head, and aim your knee outward and away from the body. Then lower the leg while straightening the knee, pointing the toes down, and bringing the leg across the opposite leg. This movement will be a combination of up and out and down and across (figure 9.25, *a-c*). Repeat 8 to 10 times, then change sides and repeat.

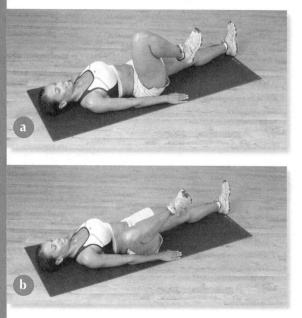

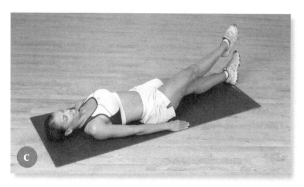

Figure 9.25 **Hip-knee-ankle, Diagonal two:** *(a)* **heel to buttock,** *(b)* **knee pointing outward, and** *(c)* **toes down and across.**

Closed Chain (Weight Bearing)

Star Balance Activities

Stand in the middle of an imaginary eight-point star, one foot in the center, and point the other foot to each point of the star, coming back to the center between each motion.

1. Straight out forward
2. Diagonally forward to the right
3. Sideways away from the body
4. Diagonally backward to the right
5. Straight backward
6. Diagonally forward to the left
7. Sideways across the body
8. Diagonally backward to the left (figure 9.26)

Repeat on the other leg.

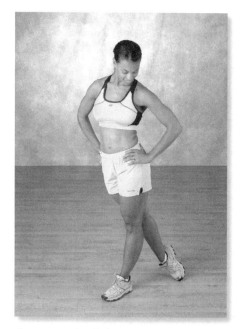

Figure 9.26 **Star balance.**

Partial Squats

Stand with your back to the wall (you may have a stability ball between you and the wall) and a smaller ball or a pillow between the knees, with your feet shoulder-width apart. Slowly slide down the wall, bending your knees about 45 degrees, then slowly straighten to your starting position (figure 9.27, *a* & *b*). Repeat 8 to 10 times.

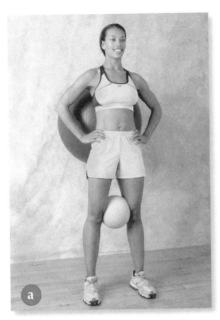 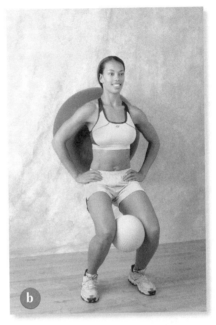

Figure 9.27 **Partial squats:** *(a)* **start,** *(b)* **finish.**

Modified Lunges

Standing, step forward with your right foot and shift your weight onto that forward foot while bending your left knee toward the ground (without touching it). Step back to your starting position, then step out with your left foot, bending your right knee toward the ground. Continue alternating and repeat 8 to 10 times on each side (figure 9.28).

Hamstring Curls

While standing and holding on to a counter or the back of a chair, slowly bring your right heel up to your buttock, then back down. Repeat 8 to 10 times. Repeat with your other leg (figure 9.29).

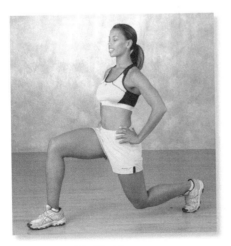 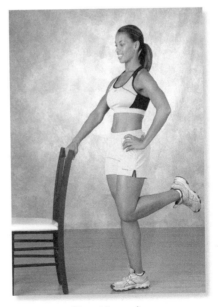

Figure 9.28 **Modified lunge.**

Figure 9.29 **Hamstring curls.**

LOWER BODY CONDITIONS

Bridging

Lying on your back, bend both knees and place feet flat on the mat. Push your buttocks and low back off the ground, keeping the rest of the trunk on the ground. Slowly lower back to your starting position, then repeat 8 to 10 times (figure 9.30).

Mule Kicks

While down on your hands and knees, keep your low back flat and gently kick the left leg back, trying to straighten the leg out behind you. Slowly come back to the starting position. Alternating legs, repeat 8 to 10 times on each side (figure 9.31).

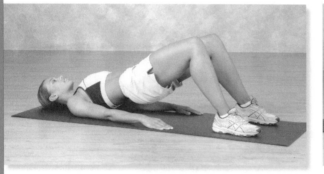

Figure 9.30 **Bridging.**

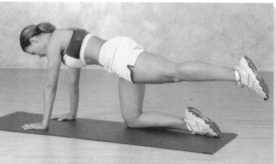

Figure 9.31 **Mule kicks.**

SUPPLEMENTAL ACTIVITIES

1. Apply ice to the affected area frequently to help control inflammation and pain.
2. Hip abduction-adduction machines (seated): If you have access to gym equipment, using the hip abduction and adduction machines will be helpful.

PRECAUTIONS

1. Avoid sitting on your wallet or other objects in your back pocket.
2. When walking up hills, concentrate on staying upright; do not bend forward.
3. Watch your foot position on the ground as you walk. The foot should point straight ahead, not be turned in or out.

Patellar Tendinitis

This condition, also called jumper's knee, is usually the result of overuse. Pain is most often felt at the bottom of the kneecap but may also occur elsewhere around the knee.

Some other conditions that have similar symptoms are patellar bursitis, patellofemoral syndrome, crepitus, and chondromalacia. These injuries may occur with direct trauma, as in falling onto the knee or banging it on something, but usually are the result of more long-term causes including tight or imbalanced muscles, sitting for excessive periods, or knees bent in abnormal positions.

After identifying the problem, your physician has several choices for care, which may include rest, nonsteroidal anti-inflammatory medications, knee braces or straps, physical therapy, or surgery as a last resort.

The condition may be further complicated by other factors such as instability or poorly aligned joints from tight muscles. These factors may prevent you from resolving your pain with a home exercise program. However, these exercises, if done correctly, will not cause further injury to your knees and should improve your symptoms, even if they don't resolve them completely.

Obviously, if your condition is worsening over time while you are trying these exercises, you should stop the activities and see your medical provider.

STRETCHES

These activities should not cause pain, but should allow for gentle increases in mobility and greater use of your knees.

1. Quadriceps, pages 55-57
2. Psoas, pages 59-60
3. Hamstrings, pages 39-41
4. Gastrocnemius, pages 62-63
5. Soleus, pages 63-64
6. Hip abductors, pages 48-50

STRENGTHENING EXERCISES

You can make these activities more challenging by adding the use of an elastic band or tubing or light weights. Resistance should be added only when the joint can be moved without increased pain.

Open Chain (Non-Weight Bearing)

Short Arc Quads (SAQs)

Lie on your back or sit with a pillow under the affected knee. Slowly straighten the lower leg, hold for 3 to 5 seconds, and slowly lower. Repeat 8 to 10 times (figure 9.32, a & b). Repeat on the other leg.

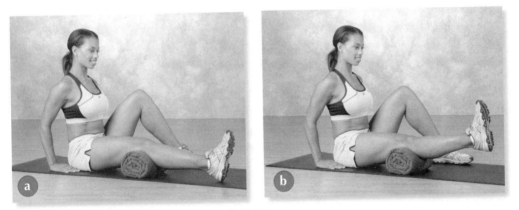

Figure 9.32 **Short arc quads (SAQs):** *(a)* **start,** *(b)* **finish.**

Straight Leg Raises—All Four Directions

Flexion: Lie on your back with both legs straight or your left knee bent, with the right foot flat on the mat. Lift your right leg upward, hold (1-2 seconds), and lower slowly. Breathe normally and repeat 8 to 10 times. Change leg positions and repeat on the other side (see figure 9.21 on p. 165).

Abduction-adduction: Lie on your back with your left leg straight out and your right knee bent, with the right foot flat on the mat. Lift your left leg up and bring it out away from your midline, hold (1-2 seconds), and slowly pull back in toward the middle. Breathe normally and repeat 8 to 10 times. Change leg positions and repeat on the other side (see figure 9.22 on p. 165).

Extension: Lie on your stomach, with your legs out straight. Lift your right leg upward, keeping it straight, hold (1-2 seconds), and lower slowly. Breathe normally and repeat 8 to 10 times. Repeat on the other side (see figure 9.23 on p. 165).

Hip-Knee-Ankle Combination PNF Diagonals

You may use ankle weights to give a little resistance for either direction of movement.

Diagonal One

Lie on your back. Bring your right leg upward, bend the knee with heel to buttock, flex the ankle so the toes are pointing toward your head, and aim your right knee toward the opposite shoulder. Then lower the leg while straightening the knee, pointing the toes down, and bringing the leg outward to the side. This movement will be a combination of up and across and down and out (see figure 9.24, *a-c,* on p. 165). Repeat 8 to 10 times, then change sides and repeat.

Diagonal Two

Lie on your back. Bring your right leg upward, bend the knee with heel to buttock, flex the ankle so the toes are pointing toward your head, and aim the knee outward away from the body. Then lower the leg while straightening the knee, pointing the toes down, and bringing the leg across the opposite leg. The movement will be a combination of up and out and down and across (see figure 9.25, *a-c,* on p. 166). Repeat 8 to 10 times, then change sides and repeat.

Closed Chain (Weight Bearing)

Star Balance Activities

Stand in the middle of an imaginary eight-point star, one foot in the center, and point the other foot to each point of the star, coming back to the center between each motion.

1. Straight out forward
2. Diagonally forward to the right
3. Sideways away from the body
4. Diagonally backward to the right
5. Straight backward
6. Diagonally forward to the left
7. Sideways across the body
8. Diagonally backward to the left (see figure 9.26 on p. 166)

Repeat on the other leg.

Partial Squats

Stand with your back to the wall (you may have a stability ball between you and the wall) and a pillow between the knees, with your feet shoulder-width apart. Slowly slide down the wall, bending your knees about 45 degrees, then slowly straighten to your starting position (see figure 9.27, *a-b,* on p. 167). Repeat 8 to 10 times.

Modified Lunges

Standing, step forward with your right foot and shift your weight onto that forward foot while bending your left knee toward the ground (without touching). Step back to your starting position, then step out with your left foot, bending your right knee toward the ground. Continue alternating and repeat 8 to 10 times on each side (see figure 9.28 on p. 167).

Hamstring Curls

While standing and holding on to a counter or the back of a chair, slowly bring your right heel up to your buttock, then back down. Repeat 8 to 10 times. Repeat with your other leg (see figure 9.29 on p. 167).

SUPPLEMENTAL ACTIVITIES

1. Apply ice to the affected area frequently to help control inflammation and pain.
2. Hip abduction-adduction machines (seated): If you have access to gym equipment, using the hip abduction and adduction machines will be helpful.

PRECAUTIONS

1. Avoid bending the knee into pain.
2. Braces should be used only for stability; long-term wear may weaken the knee.
3. Watch your foot position on the ground as you walk. The foot should point straight ahead, not be turned in or out.

Achilles Tendinitis

Achilles tendinitis is inflammation and swelling on the tendon, with pain usually localized, not radiating. This condition typically results from starting a new running activity or overdoing any running activity in a relatively short period of time. Also, trauma, such as from stepping into a hole or misstepping on a staircase, can cause this area to become inflamed. Once inflamed, this tendon normally takes a long time to settle down because the foot never gets rest unless we are off our feet completely for some period of time.

Some other conditions with similar pain are Achilles bursitis, some foot and heel conditions, and calf strain.

After identifying the problem, your physician has several choices for care, such as rest, nonsteroidal anti-inflammatory medications, stretching, massage therapy, physical therapy, cortisone injection, or walking boot or cast, but seldom surgery.

The condition may be further complicated by other factors such as ankle or knee instability, cartilage damage, or bone spurs. These factors may prevent you from resolving your pain with a home exercise program. However, these exercises, if done correctly, will not cause further injury to your calf or ankle and should improve your symptoms, even if they don't resolve them completely.

Plantar Fasciitis

This condition is inflammation of the fascia on the bottom of the foot, characterized by pain, especially for the first few steps when getting out of bed in the morning or after sitting for a period of time. Plantar fasciitis usually results from starting a new running activity or overdoing any running activity in a relatively short period of time. Trauma, such as from misstepping on a staircase, can also cause this area to become inflamed. Aging also plays an interesting, if frustrating, role. The fascia has little ability to stretch; and as we age, the muscles in the foot and calf weaken, allowing the arch to fall and thus stressing the fascia. Once inflamed, the bottom of the foot normally takes a long time to settle down because the foot never gets rest unless we are off our feet completely for some period of time.

Some other conditions with similar pain are heel spurs, painful arch, and posterior tibialis tendinitis.

Several modalities may be employed by your doctor, such as rest, nonsteroidal anti-inflammatory medications, stretching, massage therapy, physical therapy, heel lifts, cortisone injection, or a walking boot or cast, but seldom surgery.

The condition may be further complicated by other factors such as foot or ankle instability or bone spurs. These factors may prevent you from resolving your pain with a home exercise program. However, these exercises, if done correctly, will not cause further injury to your foot or ankle and should improve your symptoms, even if they don't resolve them completely.

Obviously, if your condition is worsening over time while you are trying these exercises, you should see your medical provider.

STRETCHES

These activities should not cause pain, but should allow for gentle increases in mobility and greater use of the feet and ankles.

LOWER BODY CONDITIONS

STRENGTHENING EXERCISES

You can make these activities more challenging by adding the use of an elastic band or tubing or light weights. Resistance should be added only when the joint can be moved without increased pain.

Calf Raises and Toe Raises

While sitting with both feet flat on the floor, lift the heels off the floor, keeping the balls of the feet and the toes on the floor. Slowly lower your heels, shift your weight to the heels, and lift your toes and the balls of your feet off the floor. To increase the difficulty, do these standing. Repeat 8 to 10 times (figure 9.33, *a* & *b*).

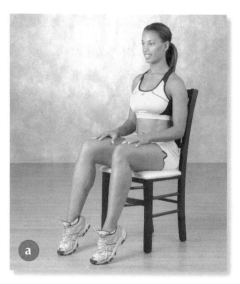
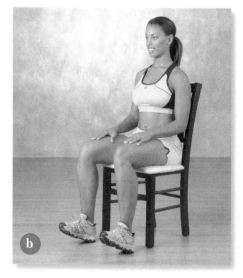

Figure 9.33 **Calf and toe raises:** *(a)* **calf raises,** *(b)* **toe raises.**

Towel Crunches

Place a small towel on a flat, smooth surface (wood or tile floor); put your foot on top and attempt to squeeze the towel with your toes and pick it up. Repeat 8 to 10 times on each side (figure 9.34).

Ankle Strengthening

(May be done sitting or lying down; repeat each motion 8-10 times.)

Dorsiflexion: Bring your toes and forefoot up toward your head.

Plantarflexion: Point the toes downward ("step on the gas").

Inversion: Turn the foot inward, trying to see the sole of your foot.

Eversion: Turn the foot outward, trying to hide the sole of the foot.

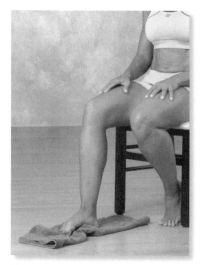

Figure 9.34 **Towel crunches.**

PNF Patterns

(Repeat each 8-10 times.)

Ankle, Diagonal One

While sitting or supine, move your foot only and bring toes up and inward, then down and outward (trying to point with the big toe) (figure 9.35, *a* & *b*).

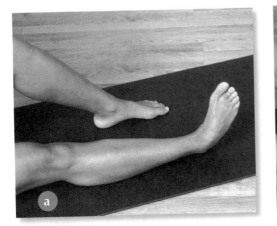 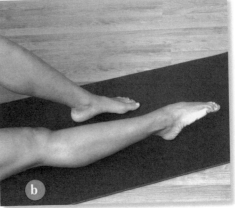

Figure 9.35   **Ankle, Diagonal one:** *(a)* **start,** *(b)* **finish.**

Ankle, Diagonal Two

While sitting or supine, move your foot only and bring the toes up and outward, then down and inward (trying to point with the big toe) (figure 9.36, *a* & *b*).

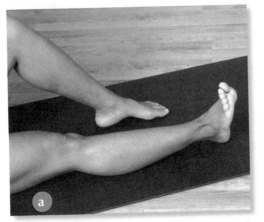 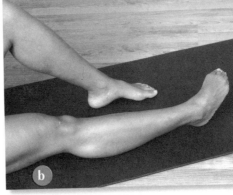

Figure 9.36   **Ankle, Diagonal two:** *(a)* **start,** *(b)* **finish.**

SUPPLEMENTAL ACTIVITIES

1. Walking on toes and heels: Actually walk on your toes for a distance, then try to walk on the heels.
2. Foot alphabet: Use your foot to write every letter of the alphabet in capital letters.

PRECAUTIONS

1. Avoid overstretching into pain.
2. Use a heel lift for a short time to reduce the pull on the calf and foot.

LOWER BODY CONDITIONS

GLOSSARY

abduction—Moving a limb away from the midline of the body, as in raising the arm horizontally.

adduction—Moving a limb toward the midline of the body, as in lowering the raised arm from a horizontal position.

adhesion—A fibrous band of scar tissue that binds together tissues that are usually separate.

agonist muscle—The muscle that contracts to move a body part.

antagonist muscle—The muscle that opposes the agonist, stretching as the agonist contracts.

anterior—Toward, located on, or near the front of the body.

axilla—The hollow under the arm, that is, the armpit.

concentric contraction—A voluntary contraction in which the muscle shortens as it works.

crossed syndrome—A condition, described by Vladimir Janda, in which groups of hypertonic muscles neurologically inhibit their antagonists, leading to specific postural imbalance patterns.

distal—Situated farthest from a point of reference such as a muscle attachment or a bony landmark.

dorsiflexion—Bending the foot upward.

eccentric contraction—A voluntary contraction in which the muscle resists while being lengthened by an outside force; also referred to as "negative work."

eccentric stress—The tension found in a muscle that is habitually eccentrically contracted in response to hypertonicity in its antagonist.

eversion—Turning the foot so that the sole faces outward.

extension—Movement at a joint that increases the joint angle and shifts the parts farther apart, as in straightening the elbow.

flexion—Movement at a joint that decreases the joint angle and shifts the parts so that they are closer together, as in bending the elbow.

glenoid fossa—The concave depression in the scapula that holds the head of the humerus to form the shoulder joint.

Golgi tendon organ (GTO)—A stretch receptor found in the tendon and at the myotendinous junction of skeletal muscle, believed to monitor the tension on a tendon.

horizontal abduction—Movement of the arm away from the midline of the body, beginning with the arm at shoulder level, as in using the right arm to draw a curtain from left to right.

horizontal adduction—Movement of the arm toward the midline of the body, beginning with the arm at shoulder level, as in using the right arm to open a curtain from right to left.

hyperextension—Movement of a joint beyond its normal position of extension, as in locking the knees back during standing.

hypertonic—Referring to a muscle that maintains a higher than normal level of concentric contraction, causing it to be short and tight.

inverse stretch reflex—*See* stretch reflex.

inversion—Turning the foot so that the sole faces inward.

isolytic contraction—An isotonic, eccentric contraction performed with the intent of stretching and breaking down fibrotic tissue.

isometric contraction—A voluntary muscle contraction during which no movement occurs.

isotonic contraction—A voluntary muscle contraction in which the muscle shortens and joint motion results.

lateral—Away from the midline.

medial—Toward the midline.

myotatic stretch reflex—*See* stretch reflex.

plantarflexion—Bending the foot downward.

posterior—Toward, located on, or near the rear of the body.

postisometric relaxation (PIR)—The reduction in muscle tone following an isometric contraction.

pronation—Turning the forearm so the hand faces downward, as in palming a basketball.

prone—Lying on the stomach, with the face down.

proprioception—Perception of spatial orientation and movement derived from sensory receptors within the body.

proximal—Situated nearest to a point of reference such as a muscle attachment or a bony landmark.

range of motion—The amount of movement available at a joint, usually expressed in degrees.

reciprocal innervation (reciprocal inhibition)—A reflex loop mediated by the muscle spindles. When a muscle contracts, reciprocal inhibition may simultaneously inhibit the opposing muscle. This allows movement to occur around a joint.

rotation—The movement of a bone around its long axis.

soft tissue barrier—The point at which soft tissue offers mild resistance to further stretching. The soft tissue barrier is the starting point for most facilitated stretches.

stretch reflex—A shortening reaction to stretch that helps protect muscles and joints from injury due to over-stretching or excessive strain. In the myotatic stretch reflex, when a muscle lengthens too quickly or too far, proprioceptors called muscle spindles, located in the belly of the muscle, are stimulated and reflexively cause the muscle to contract. The inverse stretch reflex (also called autogenic inhibition) has the opposite effect. It causes the muscle to relax in response to excessive loading of the tendons or because of excessive tension in the muscle.

supinate—To turn the forearm so the hand faces upward, as in holding a bowl of soup.

supine—Lying on the back, with the face upward.

synovial fluid—Lubricating fluid secreted by the membrane that lines joints and tendon sheaths.

target muscle—The muscle to be stretched.

REFERENCES

Anderson, B. 2000. *Stretching: 20th anniversary.* Bolinas, CA: Shelter.

Beaulieu, J.E. 1981. Developing a stretching program. *Physician and Sportsmedicine* 9 (11): 59-69.

Chaitow, L. 2001. *Muscle energy techniques,* 2nd ed. New York: Churchill Livingstone.

Chalmers, G. 2002. Do Golgi tendon organs really inhibit muscle activity at high force levels to save muscles from injury, and adapt with strength training? *Sports Biomech.* 1:239-249.

Chalmers, G. 2004. Re-examination of the possible role of the Golgi tendon organ and muscle spindle reflexes in proprioceptive neuromuscular facilitation stretching. *Sports Biomech.* 3:159-183.

Cornelius, W.L., and K. Craft-Hamm. 1988. Proprioceptive neuromuscular facilitation flexibility techniques: Acute effects on arterial blood pressure. *Physician and Sportsmedicine* 16 (4): 152-161.

Grant, K.E. 1997. Tender loving care for dancer's legs. *Tactalk* 22 (1) 6-97: 1-5.

Holt, L.E. 1976. *Scientific stretching for sport (3-S).* Halifax, Nova Scotia: Sport Research.

Hultborn, H. 2001, State-dependent modulation of sensory feedback. *J Physiol* 533 (1): 5-13.

Janda, V. 1983. *Muscle function testing.* London: Butterworths.

Lewit, K. 1999. *Manipulative therapy in rehabilitation of the motor system,* 3rd ed. London: Butterworths.

Liebenson, C. 1996. *Rehabilitation of the spine: A practitioner's manual.* Baltimore: Williams & Wilkins.

Mattes, A. 2000. *Active isolated stretching: The Mattes method.* Sarasota, FL: Author.

Moore, M.A., and R.S. Hutton. 1980. Electromyographic investigation of muscle stretching techniques. *Medicine and Science in Sports and Exercise* 12: 322-329.

Murphy, D.R. (1994). Dynamic range of motion training: An alternative to static stretching. *Chiropractic Sports Medicine* 8: 59-66.

Myers, T. 1998. Poise: Psoas-piriformis balance. *Massage Magazine* 72 (March/April): 72-83.

Myers, T. 2001. *Anatomy trains.* London: Churchill Livingstone.

Sherrington, C. 1947. *The integrative action of the nervous system,* 2nd ed. New Haven, CT: Yale University Press.

Surburg, P.R. 1981. Neuromuscular facilitation techniques in sports medicine. *Physician and Sportsmedicine* 9 (9): 115-127.

Wilmore, J.H., and D.L. Costill, 2004. *Physiology of Sport and Exercise,* 3rd ed. Champaign, IL: Human Kinetics.

Voss, D., M. Ionta, and B. Myers. 1985. *Proprioceptive neuromuscular facilitation,* 3rd ed. Philadelphia: Harper & Row.

INDEX

Note: The italicized *f* following page numbers refers to figures.

ABOUT THE AUTHORS

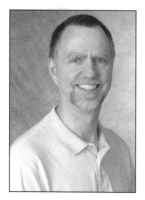

Robert McAtee

Robert McAtee, BA, LMT, CSCS, C-PT has been a massage therapist since 1981, specializing in sport and orthopedic massage therapy. Since 1988 he has maintained an active, international sport massage practice in Colorado Springs, Colorado.

McAtee received his massage training at the Institute for Psycho-Structural Balancing (IPSB) in Los Angeles and San Diego (1981-82) and through the Sports Massage Training Institute (SMTI) in Costa Mesa, CA (1986). He holds a BA in Psychology from California State University (1974), is Nationally Certified in Therapeutic Massage and Bodywork (1992), is a Certified Strength and Conditioning Specialist (1998), and an ACE-certified personal trainer (2006).

McAtee regularly presents workshops on facilitated stretching, massage, and soft-tissue injury care nationally and internationally. For more information, please contact him at: Pro-Active Massage Therapy; 1119 N. Wahsatch Ave., Suite 1; Colorado Springs, CO 80903, USA; Tel: 719-475-1172; Website: www.stretchman.com.

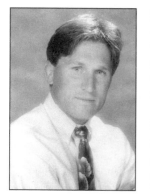

Jeff Charland

Jeff Charland, PT, ATC, CSCS, GDMT, was a 1983 graduate of the University of Wisconsin at Madison physical therapy program, where he also competed as a varsity wrestler on a scholarship. Beginning in 1987, Charland lectured in the areas of sports medicine, rehabilitation, and assessment and treatment of neural tissue disorders. He was a team trainer and traveled internationally with the U.S. Judo and U.S. Wrestling Federations' national and Olympic teams.

Charland completed the graduate program in manipulative therapy at Curtin University in Perth, Western Australia, under the direction of Bob Elvey, a world-renowned physiotherapist. He was a certified athletic trainer through the National Athletic Trainers' Association (NATA) and a Certified Strength and Conditioning Specialist (CSCS) through the NSCA. In 1997, he earned a certification in Active Release Techniques (ART). He also served as director of a sports physical therapy clinic in Colorado Springs, Colorado.

Charland passed away during the preparation of this third edition.

ABOUT THE CONTRIBUTOR

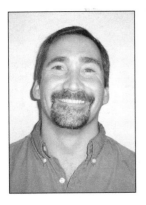

David Charland

David Charland, PT, ATC, is a 1998 graduate of the University of Health Sciences in Antigua physical therapy program. He earned a degree in Physical Education and Food, Science and Nutrition from the University of Rhode Island in 1993.

Charland received his Athletic Training Certification through the National Athletic Trainers' Association (NATA) in 1993.

DVD MENU

Section I: Introduction

Section II: Diagonal Patterns

Free Movement
D1 Pattern, Arm
D2 Pattern, Arm
D1 Pattern, Leg
D2 Pattern, Leg

Strengthening With Elastic Band
D1 Arm Flexion
D1 Arm Extension
D2 Arm Flexion
D2 Arm Extension
D1 Leg Flexion
D1 Leg Extension
D2 Leg Flexion
D2 Leg Extension

Section III: Partner Stretches

Lower Extremity
SINGLE-PLANE STRETCHES
Hamstrings, Straight Leg
Hamstrings, Bent Knee
Gluteus Maximus
Piriformis, Supine
Piriformis, Prone
Hip Abductors
Hip Adductors
Quadriceps
Psoas
Gastrocnemius
Soleus
Tibialis Anterior
Peroneals (Evertors)
Posterior (Invertor)
SPIRAL STRETCHES
Soccer Kick Stretch
Toe-Off Stretch
Snowplow Stretch

Upper Extremity
SINGLE-PLANE STRETCHES
Subscapularis Stretch
Infraspinatus and Teres Minor
Serratus Anterior
Rhomboids and Middle Trapezius
Pectoralis Minor
Pectoralis Major
Triceps
Wrist and Finger Flexors
Wrist and Finger Extensors
Forearm Supinator
Forearm Pronators
SPIRAL STRETCHES
Draw Sword
Sheath Sword
Grab Seat Belt
Fasten Seat Belt

Neck
Upper Trapezius
Sternocleidomastoid
Scalenes

Trunk
Trunk Rotators
Quadratus Lumborum
Latissimus Dorsi

Section IV: Self-Stretches

Lower Extremity
SINGLE-PLANE STRETCHES
Hamstrings With Stretching Strap
Gluteus Maximus
Piriformis, Supine
Piriformis, Sitting
Hip Abductors Sitting
Hip Adductors Standing
Quadriceps
Psoas
Gastrocnemius With Stretching Strap
Soleus
Tibialis
Peroneals (Evertors)
Tibialis Posterior (Invertor)
SPIRAL STRETCHES
Soccer Kick
Snowplow

Upper Extremity
SINGLE-PLANE STRETCHES
Subscapularis
Infraspinatus and Teres Minor
Serratus Anterior
Rhomboids and Middle Trapezius
Pectoralis Minor
Pectoralis Major
Triceps
Wrist and Finger Flexors
Wrist and Finger Extensors
Forearm Supinator
Forearm Pronators
SPIRAL STRETCHES
Draw Sword
Sheath Sword
Grab Seat Belt
Fasten Seat Belt

Neck
Upper Trapezius
Sternocleidomastoid
Scalenes

Trunk
Trunk Rotators
Quadratus Lumborum
Latissimus Dorsi

Section V: Soft Tissue Therapy Techniques
Pin-and-Stretch: Piriformis
Transverse Friction: Piriformis
Isolytic Contraction: Piriformis
Pin-and-Stretch: Subscapularis
Transverse Friction: Serratus Anterior

Section VI: Routines for Sport Activities
Running
Throwing and Racket Sports
Golf

Section VII: Credits